Take Heed

Take Heed

WATCHMAN NEE
Translated from the Chinese

"Take heed to thyself..."
1 Timothy 4.16

Christian Fellowship Publishers, Inc.
New York

ISBN 0-935008-74-8

Available from the publishers at:

11515 Allecingie Parkway
Richmond, Virginia 23235

PRINTED IN U.S.A.

TRANSLATOR'S PREFACE

"The spirit saith expressly, that in later times some shall fall away from the faith, giving heed to seducing spirits and doctrine of demons" (1 Tim. 4.1). In the light of this solemn word from Paul, therefore, a good minister of Christ Jesus ought, as the apostle had charged Timothy, to "put the bethren in mind of these things, ... for in doing this thou shalt save both thyself and them that hear thee" (vv.6,16).

At the time of the two lengthy Workers Training Sessions that were held in 1948 and 1949 at Kuling Mountain (near Foochow, China), brother Watchman Nee felt the need not only of equipping young workers to better serve the Lord but also of helping them in their spiritual life and knowledge. On the one hand, he gave talks on many weighty subjects such as Spiritual Authority, the Ministry of God's Word, etc. But on the other hand, he in addition touched on some quite elementary and yet fundamental matters such as are found in the Basic Lesson Series he gave that are instructions for new believers; and he gave many other basic presentations. For brother Nee realized that Christians can only build the weighty things upon the elementary things. If the foundation is rock-like, the building will stand; if, though, the foundation is sandy, the superstructure will collapse. How tempted we Christians are to hotly pursue after the weighty yet woefully neglect the fundamental. New believers need instruction not only in what *are* the truths; they likewise need it in what *are not*. The latter instruction is to keep us from falling, even as the former is to keep us growing and maturing.

This present volume deals exclusively with the elementary though nonetheless quite fundamental issues of the Christian life. Part One of the book, entitled "Warning and Encouragement," includes messages on the following variety of subjects: A change in Valuation, A Change of Behavior, How to Distribute Tracts, Forgive One Another, Our Attitude Towards Our Earthly Country, Waiting for the Coming of the Lord, Martyrdom, Idol Worship, and The Judaizers. All nine of these subjects were presented as messages by the author at the aforementioned Workers Training Session that was held in 1949. Notes were taken down in Chinese by a brother in the Lord, and are now being translated and published in English for the first time. To round out Part One further, two other messages, originally appearing as published articles, and entitled (1) Walk in the Will of God and (2) How to Know the Will of God, have been added. These two articles, too, are being translated and published in English for the first time.

All matters need to be understood and to become settled issues in the early years of our Christian life. Otherwise we will not be able to make much progress spiritually. They are given here with the sole purpose of helping new believers to walk in truth and love, without any intention on the part of the author to be negative in his presentation of them. May they serve as both warning and encouragement.

Finally, to complete the teaching of the present volume, twenty-seven short articles written in Chinese by Watchman Nee during 1925 and 1926 have been brought together to form Part Two, "Admonition and Discipline." They, like the contents of Part One, are being translated and published in English for the very first time as well. Though set down and published long ago in China, their value has nevertheless increased rather than decreased with the passage of time. Indeed, these articles can be invaluable to new believers at all times, they being the very admonition and discipline of the Lord. Such practical exhortations as are found in these short writings by the author are crucial to Christian growth. May the blessed Lord use them to guide His children in their heavenly pilgrimage on earth.

CONTENTS

Brief Articles Numbered 1 to 27 on the following subjects (in order of appearance): Humility, Obedience, A Righteous Christian, The Manifestation of Life, Contentment, Hiddenness, Policy, Knowledge and Judging, Quietness, A Day Like This, Never Thirsty Again, Rest, Self-proclamation, Imperfect, The Believer's Giving, Busy, Offer Secular Things, Alone, Love the Lord, Meditate on Christ, Thoughtfulness, Prayer and Desire, Holiness and Hardness, When God's Grace Manifests Itself Most, Sensitive to Sin, Read and Pray, Silent Witness.

PART ONE

WARNING AND ENCOURAGEMENT*

*For explicit information as to the sources from whence the contents of this Part were derived, see for Chapters 1 through 9 the Translator's Preface; and for chapters 10 and 11, see the footnote at the beginning of each of those two chapters. — *Translator*

1 | A Change in Valuation

Woe unto you, ye blind guides, that say, Whosoever shall swear by the temple, it is nothing; but whosoever shall swear by the gold of the temple, he is a debtor. Ye fools and blind: for which is greater, the gold, or the temple that hath sanctified the gold? And, Whosoever shall swear by the altar, it is nothing; but whosoever shall swear by the gift that is upon it, he is a debtor. Ye blind: for which is greater, the gift, or the altar that sanctifieth the gift? He therefore that sweareth by the altar, sweareth by it, and by all things thereon. And he that sweareth by the temple, sweareth by it, and by him that dwelleth therein. And he that sweareth by the heaven, sweareth by the throne of God, and by him that sitteth thereon.

Woe unto you, scribes and Pharisees, hypocrites! for ye tithe mint and anise and cummin, and have left undone the weightier matters of the law, justice, and mercy, and faith: but these ye ought to have done, and not to have left the other undone. Ye blind guides, that strain out the gnat, and swallow the camel!

> Woe unto you, scribes and Pharisees, hypocrites! for ye cleanse the outside of the cup and of the platter, but within they are full from extortion and excess. Thou blind Pharisee, cleanse first the inside of the cup and of the platter, that the outside thereof may become clean also. (Matt. 23.16–26)

Some people see the immense temple made mostly of gold and consider it to be most precious. Some see the altar with the cattle, sheep and pigeons offered upon it and think nothing of the altar yet think highly of the cattle, sheep and pigeons. Some tithe their mint, anise and cummin and have left undone the justice, mercy and faith of the law. Some are most careful in small things even to the point of straining out a gnat, and yet they swallow a camel. Some are so hasty in the use of cup and platter that they merely cleanse the outside but leave the inside full of uncleanness.

Ask any new believer how he would determine the value system of such persons as just described. Clearly the people mentioned in Matthew 23.16–26 are totally ignorant of true value. Theirs is a mistaken notion of value. As a matter of fact, the valuation of people before their conversion is invariably opposite to what is the case after their conversion experience. For in each and every believer there occurs a total change of value. What in the past he might have esteemed as precious is now no longer valuable, and what was not valuable to him before has today become precious. All who have not undergone such a change cannot be considered as

Christians. This phenomenon we would call a change in valuation.

The greater part of the Bible records this change of value. What now follow are but a few of many examples which could be cited and discussed. Let the new believers be given such light from them that they may see.

(1) "The stone which the builders rejected is become the head of the corner. This is Jehovah's doing; it is marvelous in our eyes" (Ps. 118.22–23). Here is an example of a difference in value of which we have been speaking. In the eyes of the builders mentioned the particular stone cited is unusable, and hence it is rejected. Christ is considered to be excessive; yet in the making of salvation He is taken as the chief cornerstone. A cornerstone must be smooth on at least two or three sides to be acceptable; indeed, it is often smooth on six sides. How vastly different in the spiritual realm is the valuation: a cornerstone may be rejected by the builders, but it is considered precious to God. Young believers need to be led into an understanding of this change of value. Ask them how they viewed Christ previously and how they view Him today; which is to say, bring them to see that that which was formerly worth nothing is now most worthy.

(2) "The word of the cross is to them that perish foolishness; but unto us who are saved it is the power of God" (1 Cor. 1.18). As soon as a person believes in Christ, his evaluation of things undergoes a drastic change.

(3) "Be not therefore anxious, saying, What shall we eat? or, What shall we drink? or, Wherewithal shall we be clothed? . . . But seek ye first his kingdom, and his righteousness; and all these things shall be added unto you" (Matt. 6.31,33). Our heavenly Father knows we have need of all these things; therefore, let us seek first His kingdom and His righteousness.

A poor man before his conversion thinks all the time about his daily needs; but after his faith in Christ Jesus he seeks first God's kingdom and His righteousness. For the believer who lives on earth there should be nothing more precious than the kingdom of God; for we read in Matthew 13.44 these words: "The kingdom of heaven is like unto a treasure hidden in the field; which a man found, and hid; and in his joy he goeth and selleth all that he hath, and buyeth that field." Before a person believes in the Lord, it is relatively easy for him to obtain food and clothing in times of hardship; this is because he can lie to get what he needs, since he is in no way related to the kingdom of God. But when he believes in the Lord he enters into a new environment. True, if he should still lie to get food and clothing he most surely will have his needs met, but in the process he loses God's kingdom and His righteousness. Yet what if he should *not* lie? He will gain the kingdom and righteousness, but he may lose his livelihood. How, then, should one choose? To an unbeliever, lying is nothing. Let us, however, solemnly ask a new believer how he would make his choice. It is to be hoped that he would choose the nobler part.

(4) "He that loveth father or mother more than me is not worthy of me; and he that loveth son or daughter

more than me is not worthy of me. And he that doth not take his cross and follow after me, is not worthy of me" (Matt. 10.37,38). Father, mother, wife and children should be loved when they are not in opposition to the Lord. However, under certain circumstances, a choice must be made. How, then, would you choose? Man usually chooses that which is more precious. Ask new believers whom they would choose. If this issue is not settled beforehand they will be at a loss in time of trial. Hence, the responsibility to instruct them is upon the shoulders of the leaders. Let us pose this hypothetical question to young believers: In case they have to leave father and mother and wife and children for the sake of believing in the Lord, how should they make the choice? They should choose the Lord, who died for them. They should choose to be His disciples.

(5) "What shall a man be profited, if he shall gain the whole world, and forfeit his life [soul]? or what shall a man give in exchange for his life?" (Matt. 16.26) Satan wants man's soul. How willingly people sell their soul without compensation, for they do not believe that it is worth anything. The prodigal left home not because he was invited to attend a feast. He was pulled down by the swine's husks. How worthless to an unbeliever is the soul. And yet the Lord declares that even the whole world cannot buy a man's soul. Once Satan took the Lord to an exceedingly high mountain and showed Him all the kingdoms of the world and their glory. Suppose all the world were to be given to you. How would you react? This again is a matter of value. Do you exchange your soul for the world or gain your soul and

let go the world? To lie or not to lie? Let the new believers see that honesty is more valuable than the gold and rice of the world. For the sake of keeping the soul pure, they ought to sacrifice all things. Putting new believers on the right course will help them at the outset of their experience of the change in valuation. It is our responsibility to do this.

(6) "If thy hand or thy foot causeth thee to stumble, cut if off, and cast it from thee: it is good for thee to enter into life maimed or halt, rather than having two hands or two feet to be cast into the eternal fire. And if thine eye causeth thee to stumble, pluck it out, and cast it from thee: it is good for thee to enter into life with one eye, rather than having two eyes to be cast into the hell of fire" (Matt. 18.8-9). Here once again we see the change of value. If a person does not consider the world as precious, surely he holds his body precious. When Satan tempted Job concerning his body, the latter was able to preserve his integrity (see Job 2.4-10). Here is a challenge. To preserve the body is to preserve sin; to get rid of sin demands the denial of the body. It is more serious to fall morally and spiritually than to lose the body. A believer must undergo this change in valuation. He should see the seriousness of a fall. From the outset of his new life he ought to deem sinning to be an exceedingly grave matter. To cut off a hand or to pluck out an eye bespeaks the pain involved in getting rid of sin. The sufferings are similar.

(7) "Jesus called them unto him, and said, Ye know that the rulers of the Gentiles lord it over them, and

their great ones exercise authority over them. Not so shall it be among you: but whosoever would become great among you shall be your minister; and whosoever would be first among you shall be your servant" (Matt. 20.25-27). Among the nations the rulers lord it over the people, and the great ones exercise authority over them. Yet this is not to be so among believers. Whoever wishes to be great must be a servant, and whoever wants to be first must be a bondslave. This is a change of value, a change of position. Before Christian conversion, the notion to be a ruler has great value attached to it, but the contrary notion — to be ruled over — is not something deemed valuable at all. After conversion, however, to be servants and bondslaves is considered something great and primary; whereas the desire to be rulers and great ones is now of no esteem. The position has changed because the perspective has changed. Today, the position of servants and bondslaves has become something precious: for now, the more people one *serves*, the higher and greater he is.

If in the Church people strive to be great, this is bringing the value of the world into the Church. True greatness lies in our being servants and bondslaves; and thus shall all problems in the Church be eliminated and thus shall the Church be blessed. This, however, is not an exhortation for new believers to be servants and bondslaves. Rather, it is to show the change of value that must take place so as to make the new believers willing to take the lower place. A change of value will enable them to see true greatness. Accordingly, the central thought of Christianity is a change in valuation. And such is the way of the Church.

(8) "If thou return to the Almighty, thou shalt be built up, if thou put away unrighteousness far from thy tents. And lay thou thy treasure in the dust, and the gold of Ophir among the stones of the brooks; and the Almighty will be thy treasure, and precious silver unto thee. For then shalt thou delight thyself in the Almighty, and shalt lift up thy face unto God. Thou shalt make thy prayer unto him, and he will hear thee; and thou shalt pay thy vows. Thou shalt also decree a thing, and it shall be established unto thee; and light shall shine upon thy ways" (Job. 22.23–28). The verses from verse 24 onward are based on that which is said in verse 23. The treasure and the gold mentioned here are related to the "unrighteousness" cited in verse 23. We are instructed to cast our treasure upon the dust and our gold among the stones of the brooks. Why? In order that unrighteousness may be dealt with, in order that one may delight himself in the Lord. This again is a change in valuation.

As you stand at the threshold of temptation, will you choose treasure and gold or will you choose the Lord? Herein lies the difference between those who belong to God and those who do not belong to God. All who are the Lord's will choose to delight in Him. And as the very first result, He will hear your prayer. If, though, you choose treasure and gold, your prayer will not be heard by God. Second, whatever you decide to do He will establish for you, because He is pleased with your decision and choice. Third, light shall shine upon your way. There will be light upon each of your steps.

Sooner or later, new believers must be delivered from

their old environments. Ask them how they would make their choice. They ought to choose the righteousness of God and cast away treasure and gold. The value of righteousness far exceeds that of all other things. It is a mistake to lay a heavy load upon new believers without presenting to them this change in valuation. Then let these Christians discard the cheaper things such as gold and silver and consider as treasure the most valuable things such as faithfulness, joy and prayer.

(9) "By faith, Moses, when he was grown up, refused to be called the son of Pharaoh's daughter; choosing rather to share ill treatment with the people of God, than to enjoy the pleasures of sin for a season; accounting the reproach of Christ greater riches than the treasures of Egypt: for he looked unto the recompense of reward" (Heb. 11.24–26). Here is shown the change of value in respect of pleasures and reproach. Moses understood the pleasures of sin. Yet, he considered suffering with the people of God to be most precious. He could have enjoyed the pleasures of sin, for he was a person of wealth, position and influence. Nevertheless, he refused to be called the son of Pharaoh's daughter because he counted the reproach of Christ greater riches than all the treasures of Egypt. He saw clearly the change of value. He was willing to endure any harm or reproach, for he looked to the greater recompense of reward.

(10) "Howbeit what things were gain to me, these have I counted loss for Christ. Yea verily, and I count all things to be loss for the excellency of the knowledge

of Christ Jesus my Lord: for whom I suffered the loss of all things, and do count them but refuse, that I may gain Christ" (Phil. 3.7–8). Here we see that Paul had also experienced a change in the valuation of things. What he had previously counted gain to himself, he now counts as loss for the sake of Christ. How could you force Paul to enjoy things that were now loss to him? He counted all things as loss, even refuse, for the excellency of knowing and serving the Lord Jesus Christ. He reckoned Jesus, whom God had established Lord and Christ, to be most precious. Hence he was willing to cast off all things as refuse that he might gain Him.

The Lord Jehovah is quoted in the latter part of Jeremiah 15.19 as having declared: "if thou take forth the precious from the vile, thou shalt be as my mouth." Unless you and I have settled this matter of value, none of us can be used by God. He requires us to differentiate between the precious and the vile. This indicates the importance of knowing a change of value.

2 | A Change of Behavior

One of the difficulties new believers face is that of being easily irritated. Upon their receiving grace, there ought to be a change in behavior and character—of which one facet should be a change in temper. If a person has believed in the Lord for a number of years and yet his temper has remained the same as before, he will have no testimony towards the world nor in the Church. He should undergo a change in the matter of his temper right after he believes.

Let us tell new believers that as Christians their lives ought to manifest certain characteristics. One, *to love one another:* "A new commandment I give unto you, that ye love one another; even as I have loved you, that ye also love one another" (John 13.34). Two, *to be meek:* "Blessed are the meek: for they shall inherit the earth" (Matt. 5.5); "behold, thy King cometh unto thee ... riding upon an ass" (Zech. 9.9). This is meekness. Three, *to be self-denying.* "If any man would come after me," says the Lord, "let him deny himself" (Matt. 16.24). He does not say, "let him build himself up," but, "let him deny himself." Four, *to be patient.* Believers ought to be patient amidst whatever life situation presents itself (see James 1.2–4). Five, *to be joyful.* New believers ought to rejoice in the Lord, and they should never allow anything to destroy that joy (see Phil. 4.4). Six, *to be at peace:* "the peace of God, which passeth all understanding, shall guard your hearts and your thoughts in Christ Jesus" (Phil. 4.7). Seven, *to be lowly:* "I am meek and lowly in heart," says the Lord (Matt. 11.29). The word here is "lowly" and not "lofty."

Let us present all these qualities to new believers, and then explain each one of them in relation to their temper. For example, (1) where there is love, there will be no irritation. No matter who the person is, it is the Lord's command that we should love. It is impossible to love and to lose one's temper at the same time. We live to love. (2) The Lord commands us to be meek, for He himself is so. By being gentle and tender, we are able to comfort others. If we are meek in both attitude and conduct we cannot be hot-tempered. Temper is the rudest of all emotions, while meekness is the most delicate. How can we be reckoned as meek before God if we display a bad temper? (3) The Lord calls us to deny ourselves, to be willing to be defrauded, to cast aside our own self, to never speak for our rights, and to learn to endure all things. No matter how we are treated we will not lose our temper. God's children ought to deny the self. (4) Show new believers the need of patience. Be patient in all things. Sometimes we are truly treated unreasonably, but love will not be irritated. Whatever the Lord has arranged for us, let us be patient and not be angered by it. (5) God has given us a life of always rejoicing (see again Phil. 4.4). So, in a believer's life, there is no place for wrath. Always rejoice in the Lord. (6) The same is true in respect of peace. There is nothing that can disturb our inward peace. Our thoughts and hearts are guarded from attack, thus keeping us away from being provoked (see again Phil. 4.7). (7) As children of God we are the humblest of all men. Temper and lowliness are incompatible. He who loses his temper is not lowly in heart. May we follow the lowly Christ and walk the lowly path.

Let new believers learn not to be angry. Listen to what the Lord says: "I say unto you, that every one who is angry with his brother shall be in danger of the judgment" (Matt. 5.22). Anger and hot temper are inconsistent with Christian living. Probably, temper uncontrolled is the greatest problem to most believers, and it is something that needs to be dealt with in the early stage of a new convert's life. Why is there temper? This matter must first be solved and clearly settled *in us* before we can help *our brethen* and lead them in a straight path.

By way of providing a fundamental answer to this question of why temper, let me say at the outset that temper is not a *disease* but a *symptom* of something. Though it is a serious problem among God's children, it nonetheless occupies a very small place in the Scriptures. The Bible seems to pay little attention to temper, perhaps because it is only a symptom. Let me explain. A man has appendicitis. High fever is a symptom. Due to this physical malady, there is such a symptom as fever. Yet it would be useless simply to treat the symptom.

But by removing the appendix the high fever will automatically subside. Likewise, therefore, let us keep in mind that temper is but a symptom of something deeper, which is why the Bible pays little attention to it. We must see that there is a spiritual disease that brings forth bad temper.

"Even so reckon ye also yourselves to be dead unto sin, but alive unto God in Christ Jesus" (Rom. 6.11). It would be futile to think of this verse after our temper has already been provoked to anger. No, this passage of Scripture is for the healing of the *source* of the disease. And this source that has caused the manifestation of bad temper is surely related to self. The *self* in the believer must be dealt with first. And as the self is dealt with, the problem of temper shall be solved.

Let us look at the various aspects of self in relation to this matter of temper: (1) *Subjectiveness.* Many are very subjective. They consider their self as all-important. They are used to pushing through to the forefront their own opinions. If they meet with any disapproval or disagreement, they will burst out with a display of bad temper. The root of the disease lies in their subjective view. Were they under the discipline of the Lord, they would pray, "O Lord, this is Your hand. I submit." Then that one is unable to lose his temper. As our self is dealt with, the temper shall be smitten and destroyed; furthermore, it will become easy to submit.

(2) *Pride.* This is an esteeming of oneself too highly—the considering of oneself as superior to and distinguished from other people. All the proud ones look for exaltation. They want people to lift them up.

When they encounter people who fail to recognize their worth or to acknowledge them as such, their temper is stirred. This is because their pride is hurt. And hence, the cause of temper is pride. In the case of those who have been disciplined, however, when they are despised, slandered, reproached or criticized, they will react by saying, "O Lord, this is Your dealing. I accept it because this comes from Your hand." Thus they are able to submit themselves under the mighty hand of the Lord. As they deny themselves, temper loses its power.

(3) *Self-love.* Many express love of self. They regard themselves as most important and precious among the crowd. Everything is for self. All the necessities of life are for one's own self, whether it be eating or dwelling or sleeping or whatever. Suppose some other member of the family eats what is supposedly yours, or another occupies your dwelling or even your seat. You lose your temper because you are deprived of an opportunity to exercise self-love. You are unwilling to let your self suffer. If anyone should unknowingly hurt your self-love, you naturally will break out in a bad temper. It is futile to deal with the issue of temper and not deal with the more fundamental issue of self. We live on earth by the grace and mercy of the Lord and not by our own self. We may thus encounter some provocation and still not lose our temper. On the other hand, without a dealing with self, our temper cannot be controlled.

(4) *Love of things.* Some people not only love themselves, they also love things. They have not been delivered from material things such as money and other commodities. In the event their possessions are destroyed, their temper will be raised. This is because their

love of things has been hurt. Actually, the cause for anger lies in themselves rather than in others. Brother Lawrence of long ago once struck wood, glass and a wall with his hand. Each gave off a different sound or echo. This enabled him to understand that the sound did not come from the hand but from the inherent qualities of these materials. Such is the same in the matter of man's temper. All and sundry circumstances merely touch off the temper within a person. How foolish it is to deal with temper without first dealing with self. The flaring up of temper indicates a resistance to the discipline of the Holy Spirit as well as a rejection of the arrangement of God.

(5) *Only caring about one's own affairs.* Some people like to be left quiet and alone. They have an interest only in their own affairs. They have no interest in others' affairs for the sake of the latters' welfare. Since all is for self they have no time or energy for other people. If they are sought after they feel put upon. They cannot stand to be disturbed, for they regard such as an invasion of their freedom. And the result is the rising up of anger and bad temper. Let new believers know and realize that the root of all things surrounding temper lies in their very own self.

(6) *Self-exaltation.* Some get angry because they want to exalt themselves. They do not like to see others coming up. They do not want or expect others to possess what they themselves possess. In short, they become jealous. This occurs not only in the worldly realm, it also occurs in the spiritual realm. The manifestation of such an attitude among Christians is most distasteful. In reality, such a feeling and attitude in them is not any

different from Satan's: they rejoice at seeing those whom they dislike *fall;* and in so doing, do they not manifest the same nature as Satan? But those who know God and the ways of God, they rejoice at others' *exaltation.* Jealousy must therefore be plucked out of the heart. Then temper will come under control.

Temper, then, comes out of self. How the latter needs to be dealt with in all its many facets! How much we need to learn. As we prostrate ourselves before God we shall receive light and see our true condition. Many things happen to us in a given day. Let us bow our heads and accept them, saying, "O Lord, Your ordering is the best." Many cattle and sheep do not know their herder or shepherd; they only see the rod and the staff in the latter's hands. Our looking at environments will only create disturbance—yea, even anger and bad temper. But our seeing that all is given by the Shepherd of our souls will bring in rest. Everything can be resolved if we accept the discipline of the Holy Spirit and the ordering of God. Then later on, when anger or bad temper might commence to arise, we can immediately recognize self. And quickly thereafter we shall rebound in the light.

3 | How to Distribute Tracts

Today we will talk about the distribution of tracts. In these past two or three hundred years the Church has witnessed the effectiveness of tracts well written and well distributed. Many have been saved through such literary instruments. In China the distributing of tracts has had a poor impact. This is partly because the tracts we produce are either unclear or lacking in effectiveness. We therefore hope that a discussion on this matter of tract distribution will teach good lessons for second-generation Christians.

A. *The advantages of tract distribution.* This Christian activity has many benefits: (1) Many people have trouble in speaking clearly. They may also be naturally shy. They must nevertheless open their mouths and witness for the Lord. Not because they lack eloquence can they be excused from speaking. They should still be given opportunity to speak for the Lord. Even so, some do have difficulties in speech. They may not be clear

on truth. They may be unable to tell sinners how empty
the world is, how hateful sin is, how sin deprives men
of peace, how powerful sin is, and how men can repent
and be justified. With such limitations in them they
cannot speak well, but they can certainly distribute
tracts. They can choose those which suit the needs of
their friends and relatives and then pass them out. These
literary instruments can speak more clearly than they
can; they can also present the truth much more accu-
rately. This is the first advantage — that tracts can serve
as a supplement to one's deficiency.

(2) In leading people to Christ, there is an important principle involved. Certain people are used by the
Lord to approach a certain kind of sinner. For example, it is not very fitting to send a child out to lead an
old man to Christ. It is more appropriate to send an
old person out for that task. A youth for a youth, a
nurse for a nurse, etc., etc. Ordinarily speaking, we
should approach people of the same level and gender.
It looks more natural for a sister to contact another
woman, though we acknowledge that there may be ex-
ceptions. Being a man, it is not easy for me to preach
to young women. It is hard to bridge the gap. So, a tract
becomes an excellent way.

Further, it may be difficult for a young woman to
talk to an elderly man. There are definite disadvantages.
After much prayer and receiving power from on high,
she may indeed be able to overcome the obstacles. But
such a development is exceptional. However, it involves
no such difficulties if after prayer she should respectfully present him with a tract. She could even say (if
it be the truth) that because she is a new believer she

does not know how to speak, and therefore she is giving him a tract instead. This is not expecting the tract to work for her; rather, it is a supplementary way of working. One eventually does have to learn how to open one's mouth.

(3) A tract is not influenced by affection or courtesy. In preaching the gospel from the pulpit, one can sternly talk about sin and judgment. But in witnessing one on one, there is a certain amount of courtesy and face-saving involved. You are not able to speak as frankly as you might wish. If you point out sins too personally, you may not be able to see him or her the following day. It is quite a delicate matter to speak the truth in personal conversation. But here you can give the person a tract which tells this one that we all have sinned and need to believe in Jesus. As the person reads the tract you can pray by that one's side. Then ask the person if he or she knows that he or she has sins. Thus you will not be put to much blame. We do not want to offend people in preaching the gospel, but we have to speak the truth in love. Sometimes there may be a class distinction. Give the person a tract and pray for that unbeliever. The advantage of a tract lies in its being able to speak frankly without emotional involvement.

(4) When you encounter a person who has no desire to hear the gospel but who likes to argue, then you are really put to the test. As you witness to him, do not argue even if he challenges you. It is best to give him a tract. With the latter he has no way to argue back. Oftentimes we meet relatives who thrive on argument. Respectfully present them with tracts. Then ask them the next day if they have read them and whether they

would like to have another one. Avoid direct argument. Pray for them.

(5) A tract is not bound by time and space. When we are *here,* we cannot be *there* at the same time. But a tract can do our job of witnessing without any restriction like this. Sometimes it is hard to witness to total strangers. A printed message, however, can witness at any time and to anyone anywhere. It is not restricted by time, place or person.

(6) "Cast thy bread upon the waters; for thou shalt find it after many days. ... In the morning sow thy seed, and in the evening withhold not thy hand; for thou knowest not which shall prosper, whether this or that, or whether they both shall be alike good" (Eccl. 11.1,6). Solomon said you can cast your bread upon the waters. The more you sow, the more you reap. In the spreading of the gospel, there is nothing that can exceed tracts in the amount distributed. You can sow anywhere and to any person. One brother distributed over a thousand tracts per day for two to three years. Nothing can be scattered as effortlessly as tracts. This truly is sowing a great quantity. In addition, it is so convenient. Many who are greatly used of the Lord love to distribute gospel leaflets. You do not waste your time even when walking. How regrettable if your walking time is not utilized.

(7) There is no distinction with respect to the person who distributes tracts. In preaching the gospel or in witnessing, people with gift and power seem to be able to win more to Christ, whereas people with less gift and power win fewer to Christ. This is not true in the sharing of tracts. Even a child or one who is illiterate

can give them out. So the scope of service is much wider. Anyone can do it. So long as godly people are willing to save money for the printing of tracts, men, women and children can circulate them. The work of preaching from the pulpit is limited to certain brothers and sisters. The work of distributing tracts is open to all. Let those who share tracts know that they are participating in the service of God. This is a great blessing to the Church. By doing this work their hearts will be burdened with souls as well as be turned towards the Church. There is no work so universal in its impact as the distributing of tracts.

B. *How people get saved through tracts.* In one case a tract had been distributed but was torn in two by the receiver. Another person picked up one torn half of the tract. The one word from it — "flee from the wrath to come" — caught his eyes. As a result he was saved through that very word. In another case, a certain man, as he walked, discovered a nail coming through the sole of his shoe. He found a tract on the ground, folded it and padded his shoe with it. Upon arriving home, he took out the tract and read it. The result: he got saved. Such truly is the result of casting bread upon the waters.

In England there were two men who had a clear understanding of the gospel and were used of God to save many people. One of them preached the gospel for thirty-seven years. It was common for him to preach to three to four thousand souls at open-air meetings. The other one traveled everywhere to distribute tracts. He had over a hundred different ones which he handed out in cities and villages. This work of his was most effective. Once he was on a train. The conductor called out, "Have your ticket ready." The distributor of tracts followed this up by saying, "Do you have *this* ticket?" Immediately he presented to the passengers a tract about the Ticket to Heaven. That day a number of people got saved. He was one who both printed and distributed his own tracts.

George Cutting wrote a booklet entitled "Safety, Certainty, and Enjoyment." It is very clear on salvation, and it has become next only to the Bible in the amount of circulation. Tell these stories to new believers. There were four Englishmen of differing ages greatly used by the Lord. It so happened that one had led the other to Christ and so on until all four became great soul winners. They were all saved through tracts. You have four generations here. You do not know how great can be the effectiveness of tracts.

C. *How to distribute tracts.* There are two ways of distributing tracts. One is the ordinary way of sowing, about which a few observations need to be made: (1) The tracts used must be powerful, with the ability to "catch" the "fish." Test them out if they are effective in saving souls. Then those that are effective can be used repeatedly, while those that are ineffective can be discarded. It is the same as in preaching from the pulpit. The messages which win souls can be preached elsewhere too. For preaching is for the purpose of saving souls. Some tracts produce fruits. They should be reprinted.

(2) Before distributing pray for God's blessing, that

each and every printed message will bring blessing to the people who receive them.

(3) In going out, let one be neatly dressed. Do not put on torn clothing nor dress shabbily. Be courteous. Moreover, in handing out tracts on the street do not violate the rules of the local police.

(4) Maintain a sincere attitude while sharing tracts. Do not joke nor be flippant. Do not be rude like the vagabonds. Before handing out the tract, make a bow. After he or she receives the gospel leaflet, give that person another nod of the head. In the face of abuse do not argue. Return opposition with politeness.

(5) After coming back, pray again for these tracts and their recipients. The more the prayer, the more the fruit. Ask the Lord to bless all who have received tracts. Pray that these messages of the printed page will not die out but will continue to pass from hand to hand. Pray that each time they change hands they will save souls. Pray for the longevity of the tracts.

The other way is a more special manner in the distribution of tracts (a more systematic way of delivering them). Two brothers or two sisters could be assigned to a certain street for the sharing of tracts. First pray and then distribute. Do this once a week or even more frequently. Choose the right tract for each distribution. Let each printed gospel message deal with a specific subject. After circulation pray for blessing.

There are different ways to do this. You could write the name of the head of the household on an envelope containing the tract, and then deliver it in person. This can be done for every house on the street. Or you can put a tract inside an addressed envelope and place it in the house's mail box. If someone asks what you are doing, you can reply that you are sending the glorious gospel of God's Son to that household.

Such a way of tract distribution has been highly successful in other parts of the world. Family after family has been saved.

Such a personal way of sharing tracts can be very useful and effective towards friends and relatives. Sometimes it is difficult to talk to them face to face. Choose carefully the tracts to be used—ones such as those dealing with sin, money, vanity, and so forth. Pray for blessing after these tracts have been selected. Present them with sincerity. Tell their recipients that because you are neither able to say many words nor know much yourself, therefore you are giving them these tracts to read. After delivering these tracts pray again, asking God to bless them. Thus you can easily share the gospel with them.

Distributing tracts is like fishing. You need to have the right bait. Some tracts are ineffective. If there is incorrect spelling, the tract will lose its sharpness. In God's work no carelessness can be allowed. Learn to approach a certain person with a certain word. Many are saved by the preaching about vanity. Not a few are saved through hearing of the amazing love of God. People usually know what sin really is after they have believed. Backsliders are revived by messages on sin.

To carry tracts in your pocket is commendable. A tract often opens the door for sharing the gospel. People will not feel as though they are being imposed upon.

4 | Forgive One Another

Then came Peter, and said to him [Christ], Lord, how oft
shall my brother sin against me, and I forgive him? until
seven times? Jesus saith unto him, I say not unto thee,
Until seven times; but, Until seventy times seven. Therefore is the kingdom of heaven likened unto a certain king,
who would make a reckoning with his servants. And when
he had begun to reckon, one was brought unto him, that
owed him ten thousand talents. But forasmuch as he had
not wherewith to pay, his lord commanded him to be sold,
and his wife, and children, and all that he had, and payment to be made. The servant therefore fell down and worshipped him, saying, Lord, have patience with me, and
I will pay thee all. And the lord of that servant, being
moved with compassion, released him, and forgave him
the debt. But that servant went out, and found one of
his fellow-servants, who owed him a hundred shillings;
and he laid hold on him, and took him by the throat, saying, Pay what thou owest. So his fellow-servant fell down
and besought him, saying, Have patience with me, and

I will pay thee. And he would not: but went and cast him into prison, till he should pay that which was due. So when his fellow-servants saw what was done, they were exceeding sorry, and came and told unto their lord all that was done. Then his lord called him unto him, and saith to him, Thou wicked servant, I forgave thee all that debt, because thou besoughtest me: shouldest not thou also have had mercy on thy fellow-servant, even as I had mercy on thee? And his lord was wroth, and delivered him to the tormentors, till he should pay all that was due. So shall also my heavenly Father do unto you, if ye forgive not every one his brother from your hearts. (Matt. 18.21-35)

Today we will touch on this issue of forgiving one another. How should a believer react when he is offended? He should forgive. Here are a few points to ponder on the Scripture passage just now read.*

1. At that time Peter came forward and asked, "Lord, how oft shall my brother sin against me, and

---

*The reader may wish to compare the treatment of this Scripture passage which now follows, given by the author in 1949, with a similar but shorter treatment of it which he gave a year earlier at the First Workers Training Session held at the same Conference Center on Mount Kuling outside Foochow. It can be found in translated form as the first part of the Basic Lesson that is entitled "Restore Your Brother," appearing in volume 4 of the now well-known Basic Lesson Series by Watchman Nee that is entitled *Not I But Christ* (New York: Christian Fellowship Publishers, 1974), pp. 43-45 (subhead section of the chapter noted as "The First Responsibility—Forgiveness"). — *Translator*

I forgive him? until seven times?" It is for our profit
that such a question asked has been recorded. We notice
first of all that Peter's spirit is not right; nevertheless,
we can be taught in this matter of forgiveness anyway.
Instead of how many times I should forgive a brother
who sins against me, it is far better to ask God how
many times He will forgive me my sins against Him.
If God forgives us seven times, would that be enough?
This is really an unworthy question. If I sin against God,
it is God's feelings that are hurt. I am not sensitive
enough. If my brother sins against me, my feelings are
hurt, and it is hard for me to forgive. But love seeks
not its own benefit. In asking this question, Peter is
seeking something for his own. He has been hurt, and
the cost of forgiving is his own self. Hence he asks
whether forgiving seven times is enough for him. He
considers himself to be quite generous, for he adds up
the number of times to seven. But the whole thought
is basically wrong. For he thinks that the grace of God
has a limit, though in reality it has none. Therefore,
there should also be no limit with respect to forgiving
the children of God.

"Take heed to yourselves: if thy brother sin, rebuke
him; and if he repent, forgive him. And if he sin against
thee seven times in the day, and seven times turn again
to thee, saying, I repent; thou shalt forgive him" (Luke
17.3-4). Even after your brother sins against you seven
times *in a day* and repents each time, you must forgive
him. Having heard this the apostles immediately followed
up with a prayer to the Lord, "Increase our faith" (v.5).
It appears that they could hardly believe what they had
just heard. No matter what your brother says, so long

as he says, I repent, forgive him. Do not question his honesty; if he turns back, forgive him. In Peter's question recorded in Matthew 18, however, the words, "in the day," have been omitted. Actually, in Luke's record it refers to the same person, the same situation, and the same offence as in Matthew 18. But Peter, according to Matthew's Gospel, has changed the wording, thus making the grace of forgiveness smaller and limited.

In verse 22 of Matthew 18, we find Jesus' reply to Peter as follows: "I say not unto thee, Until seven times; but, Until seventy times seven." In other words, the love and grace of God in forgiving is without limit. If we should forgive, say thirty-five times, we no doubt will become quite tense. Seventy times seven is far beyond human strength. The trial is too heavy to bear. So this power of forgiving is totally beyond man's ability. To possess such power we must seek it outside of the natural. With man it is impossible, and it is no wonder, then, that the disciples asked the Lord to increase their faith in this matter. In order to forgive we need to receive a power other than our own. According to the original text, Jesus said: "I say not unto thee, seven times." By which is meant that in forgiving, you do not count the number of times. And yet, if you *must* count, count seventy times seven!

2. In verses 23–27 the kingdom of heaven is likened by Jesus to a certain king who makes a reckoning with his servants. During the time of reckoning, a servant who owed him ten thousand talents is brought to him. In the kingdom of heaven, God shall rule over the earth just as do the kings of the earth today. Ten thousand

talents is worth about three hundred thousand ounces of gold. The amount this servant owes is so immense that it is almost incalculable. He has absolutely no way to repay this tremendous debt. Here the Lord shows us that as sinners before Him we owe Him much more than we could ever repay. Anyone who refuses to forgive forgets how great is the forgiveness he himself has received. Whoever knows the hugeness of the debt he owes is prone to be generous in forgiving his brother. But he who fails to realize the immensity of the grace he has received tends in turn to be ungracious. Here in Jesus' parable, the master commands that the debtor-servant and all he has be sold as payment. If a person commits sin he will be judged in eternity as well as in this world. Even after all is sold the debt is still not cleared. No amount of good works can ever possibly reimburse the debt.

Verse 26 tells how the servant falls down before the king and pleads for mercy, saying, "Lord, have patience with me, and I will pay thee all." He asks the lord for a little more time. He does not ask for mercy; he only asks for patience. It does not even come to his mind to ask for mercy and forgiveness. Here we see two sides: one, the long side of the servant; and two, the short side of the servant. The long side is his asking the lord for patience. In judgment he expects grace. The moment people cease from talking righteousness with God is the very time that God gives grace. It is right for men to come to God for grace. Seeking grace from God, even without the benefit of the light of the gospel, is both proper and pleasing to Him. To be conscious of his debt and to ask for mercy is precious in God's sight

Now, though, let us see the short side. The servant is not clear enough concerning the depth of his sin and debt. He is still thinking of repaying it later. He forgets that he owes *ten thousand* talents—a sum too immense ever to repay. Due to his lack of appreciating the greatness of his debt to the king, he is unable to forgive his fellow-servant. Not to say that he cannot repay his debt to the king in a lifetime, even if he had *ten* lifetimes he could still not pay back what he owes. At the time of our salvation, the sense of the sinfulness of sin is most inadequate on our part. One does not really know how great a sinner he is. Hence, there is the need of such a discovery later on, that he may ask for grace. Here in the parable, the king is moved with compassion. He pities his servant and forgives him his debt. He also sets the servant free—yet not to work for reparation but to be free indeed. Similarly, what God himself does always exceeds man's prayer. In the parable the servant pleads for patience, but the king is moved with compassion and forgives all the debt.

What is the gospel? It is God giving grace to men according to His own good pleasure. It is abundant forgiveness bestowed upon sinners, yet not according to the need of sinners but according to the riches of God. Here are some examples of this from the Scriptures: (a) The robber on the cross prayed, "Jesus, remember me when thou comest in thy kingdom." The Lord answered, "Verily I say unto thee, Today shalt thou be with me in Paradise" (Luke 23.42,43). The robber's prayer was really out of order, but the Lord's answer was according to His riches and in keeping with God's gracious character.

(b) The publican, standing afar off, dared not lift up his head but smote his breast, saying, "God, be thou merciful to me a sinner" (Luke 18.13). Mercy is the starting point of the work of God, not its termination. The Lord will most gladly spend and be spent for our souls. He said, "This man went down to his house justified" (v.14), that is to say, it was as though in God's sight he had never sinned. That is mercy!

(c) When the prodigal son came home he was thinking of saying to his father, "I have sinned against heaven, and in thy sight: I am no more worthy to be called thy son: make me as one of thy hired servants" (Luke 15.18b -19). He hoped he could convince his father and thus receive grace. He dared not expect his father to spend and be spent further for him. Yet his father—watching for his son—saw him from afar, was moved with compassion, ran, and fell on his neck, and kissed him. His father interrupted his son's pleading half-way through his prepared entreaty and ordered the servants to bring out the best things for him. Though our prayer may not be good, God's answer far exceeds our expectation. The gospel must so work till God's own heart is satisfied. For He ever bestows abundant grace and full mercy.

(d) A man who was palsied was brought on a cot to the Lord. He merely expected to be healed from his palsy, but the man received forgiveness of his sins as well. The sins which had caused his sickness were pardoned (cf. Luke 5.17–26). God dispenses grace to us according to His own knowledge.

Though the servant in Jesus' parable from Matthew does not fully understand grace, God is nonetheless delighted to be taken advantage of. Nothing pleases Him more than one's giving Him the opportunity to give grace. To the debtor it is a ten-thousand-talent debt, but to God, He is able to forgive much much more. This is the good pleasure of God.

3. In verses 28–30 we see how this servant who has been forgiven by the king now treats his fellow-servant. What is the purpose of so great a grace coming upon the servant? A person who is forgiven ought to exhibit at least a little of God's nature. He should delight in generosity, thus reflecting something of the image of the Lord. Yet after receiving such grace from his king the servant has not learned anything. He fails to touch the liberality of grace. We learned from verse 27 that he had just been forgiven, and therefore he ought to be thankful. But when he seeks out his fellow-servant who owes him a mere hundred shillings, he takes him by the throat and demands of him, "Pay what thou owest" (v. 28). His own debt to the king had come to about three hundred thousand ounces of gold, while he is owed by his fellow-servant only a hundred shillings, which is approximately three grams of gold. The difference is one million to one!

What the Lord is trying to say to Peter is that this question of forgiveness is a spiritual issue. If at the time you are saved you are filled with a sense of forgiveness, you will be full of the joy of grace, and you accordingly will love to forgive others. In asking his original question of the Lord, there is evidenced a tremendous lack in Peter's heart of the feeling of having been forgiven. Hence he himself cannot forgive. If we are filled with an overwhelming sense of having been forgiven, we will never say, "seven times." Now because Peter mentions the number seven, our Lord in response purposely chooses another number, seventy times seven—a number that can dramatically show the vast difference between the two. For when God forgives He never counts the number of times. If we keep on counting the number of times we forgive, then we are not really those who have ever counted the amount of grace we ourselves have received. Oddly enough, some do not have the consciousness of having been forgiven at all. They do not have a sense of grace received. Therefore, they are not able to forgive.

In verses 29 and 30 we ae told that the fellow-servant falls down and asks for patience. But the freed and forgiven servant will not grant patience towards his fellow-servant. Grace has not produced in him an understanding of his brother's need. He instead casts him into prison till the latter should pay what he owes. Here we have three persons, but two creditors and two debtors: the king in the parable is a creditor; the first servant is both a debtor and a creditor, and the second servant is a debtor. The Lord shows us here that the forgiven debtor ought to behave like the creditor who forgave him. The first creditor (the king) speaks words of grace and not of righteousness. But the second creditor (the servant) speaks harsh words of righteousness and not of grace. This constitutes his condemnation.

How, on the one hand, can he the forgiven debtor expect grace from his creditor and later, on the other hand, demand righteousness when he himself is a creditor? It is altogether unreasonable to ask for patience as a debtor and not to grant patience as a creditor. Peter ought to see how great the forgiveness of his sins is that he has received. He omits the phrase "in the day" in his question, and this is indeed unjustified. What is owed to the forgiven servant is but three grams of gold, which is a very insignificant amount. Is he who has been forgiven and freed by his master wrong in demanding payment from his fellow-servant? His casting the latter into prison is righteousness; nevertheless, for one who has just experienced an act of tremendous grace to so act is absolutely wrong. If we have had our sins forgiven and yet refuse to forgive others, our condemnation is certain.

4. At the end of verse 31 we see how the Lord in His parable allows the fellow-servants to speak out. They have seen what has happened and they are exceedingly sorry. Similarly, the heart of the Church is hurt too. Even seventy times seven cannot compare with ten thousand talents. How could one dare to mention "seven times"? The whole Church knows that something is wrong. And in the parable all the other servants report this sorry development to the master.

"Thou wicked servant," says the king, "I forgave thee all that debt, because thou besoughtest me: shouldest not thou also have had mercy on thy fellow-servant, even as I had mercy on thee?" (vv.31-2) Among the brethren we should speak only of forgiveness and not of righteousness. We ought to have compassion. We must not take advantage of our brothers but try our best instead to give grace. For we have ourselves received such amazing grace. The Church should be filled with forgiveness. The Lord forgives us for two reasons: one, He forgives our debt that we may be free; and two, He wants us, too, to have the power to forgive: "shouldest not thou also have had mercy on thy fellow-servant?" Everyone who has received mercy ought also to be one who shows mercy.

"Forbearing one another, and forgiving each other, if any man have a complaint against any; even as the Lord forgave you, so also do ye" (Col. 3.13). Never demand or consider righteousness. Since God does not reckon or calculate our debt, let us not be those who reckon either.

As a result the king is so angry that he delivers the unforgiving servant to the tormentors till he should pay all that is due (see v.34). In spiritual reality we are delivered into the governmental hand of God until the debt be paid. Of course, the debt being paid still points to being forgiven. We are put under discipline until we are filled with the spirit of forgiveness.

In this matter of forgiving, the Lord Jesus gives us a further word: "So shall also my heavenly Father do unto you, if ye forgive not every one his brother from your hearts" (v.35). What does this mean: "forgive . . . his brother from your hearts"? If my brother owes me three grams of gold and I find it difficult to forgive him, this proves that I do not know God. For though I myself owed three hundred thousand ounces of gold, I received forgiveness. How, then, can I be bound by three grams of gold? The incomparable liberality of the grace of forgiveness which God has bestowed upon me creates in me also a heart of superlative generosity in forgiving others. This is what forgiving a brother from the heart means. When a spirit of criticism and reckoning increases in the Church many problems arise. Let us submit ourselves under God's authority; the kingdom of heaven is full of forgiveness. Otherwise, the Church will be inundated with difficulties. To be filled with the spirit of forgiveness is to be filled with love. If that be the case, how glorious the Church will be!

5 | Our Attitude Towards Our Earthly Country*

The attitude we take towards our earthly country is an issue very important to our personal life. New believers should have dealings in this area lest they go astray.

(1) *The position of the Lord.* When the Lord Jesus was on earth He never acted as an enforcer or executor of the law, whether civil or criminal. In Luke 12.13–14 we read that two brothers asked Him to divide the inheritance for them, but He refused to comply. This was not because He opposed the dividing of an inheritance,

---

*As indicated in the Preface, this and the other first nine chapters of the present volume are the translated texts of messages which the author delivered to those assembled for the Second Workers Training Session that was convened for several months during 1949 at Mount Kuling, near Foochow, China. The readers of Watchman Nee may notice some similarities between the message now translated and published here for the first time and another message entitled "The Kingdom" which appears on pages 57–65 of Watchman Nee, *The Spirit of Judgment* (New York: Christian Fellowship

for in the Old Testament there is such a command. The question therefore lies not in whether it is right to divide an inheritance, but rather, in whether the *Lord* should do it. In John 8.3–11 the scribes and Pharisees are decribed as bringing a woman taken in adultery to Jesus and asking Him to condemn her. But the Lord stooped down and wrote with His finger on the ground. When He was repeatedly asked He lifted himself up and said to them, "He that is without sin among you, let him first cast a stone at her" (v.7). When they heard it, one by one they left. And the Lord said to her, "Neither do I condemn thee: go thy way; from henceforth sin no more" (v.11). Again, this does not mean that there should be no judgment. But the Lord has made it clear that He has not come to judge or to enforce the law. He does not engage himself in enforcing either civil or criminal law.

When Jesus was on earth His walk was as a meek and lowly Man. He never sought earthly greatness in terms of position or power. The Jewish people had wanted Him to be King on earth; they even had sought, in fact, to "take him by force to make him king"; with Jesus, however, willfully avoiding their attempt by "withdraw[ing] again into the mountain himself alone" (John 6.15). By contrast the mission of the Roman Catholic pope and his ecclesiastical Office would ap-

---

Publishers, 1984). This latter message was one of the now well-known 52 Basic Lessons which the author had presented during the convening of the very *first* Workers Training Session held on Kuling in 1948. A year later at the 1949 Session the author had a different purpose in mind which accounts for whatever differences exist between the two messages.—*Translator*

pear to be very much involved with political and other secular activities. Our Lord, however, would not touch politics; for His work was to be spiritual and not political in nature. Riding into Jerusalem on an ass, He came not in grandeur but in humility. The Jews would seek to kill Him because He said He was the Son of God. He was judged twice over. The Jewish high priest asked Him if He were the Son of God. Not having the authority to put people to death because at this time Israel was under occupation as a province of the Roman Empire, the high priest sent Jesus to the Roman governor, Pontius Pilate. Pilate, not concerned with whether Jesus was the Son of God, asked Him if He were the King of the Jews. What the Governor—as representative of the occupying Roman government—was concerned about was the possibility of a political problem developing.

How strange it is that people do not recognize who the Lord Jesus is and what was the nature of His mission on earth. They are not sure if He was a political person during His earthly walk. For the past two thousand years the world has viewed Christianity in the same way. Some advocate using religion to achieve political aims. The accusation against Jesus which had brought Him to the cross was written in three languages upon the placard placed above His head: "This is the King of the Jews" (Luke 23.38; see also John 19.19–20). Yet the Lord Jesus had no interest in politics; for did He not say, "My kingdom is not of this world"? (John 18.36) His kingdom is not to be found within the realm of the world's politics but outside that realm. Such is the position of the Lord on this vital matter.

"Jehovah saith unto my Lord, Sit thou at my right hand, until I make thine enemies thy footstool" (Ps. 110.1). Here the Father said to the Son, "Sit thou at my right hand, until I make thine enemies thy footstool." On this earth during the dispensation of grace, the Lord does not directly manage the affairs of the world. He will wait till all His enemies have become His footstool.

"Wherefore, receiving a kingdom that cannot be shaken, let us have grace, whereby we may offer service well-pleasing to God with reverence and awe" (Heb. 12.28). "Confirming the souls of the disciples, exhorting them to continue in the faith, and that through many tribulations we must enter into the kingdom of God" (Acts 14.22). In both these passages we see that the kingdom of God has no relationship to the politics of this world. God is establishing a kingdom in grace, which embraces people from all nations. This kingdom is entered through new birth. It has neither a territory nor armaments nor political structure. The command of God (which is the meaning of *this* kingdom) governs men's behavior. It is called the kingdom of the *heavens* because its position is heavenly. It does not stand at the back of any nation in the world. This kingdom rules its citizens by *spiritual,* not earthly, principles. Indeed, at the second coming of the Lord His authority shall cover the whole earth. Out of His mouth shall proceed a sharp two-edged sword, which is His word. With that He will smite the nations, and then He shall rule over them with a rod of iron (see Rev. 1.16, Eph. 6.17b, Rev. 19.15). At that time, the prayer which centuries earlier had come from the lips of the robber on the cross—

"Jesus, remember me when thou comest in thy kingdom"—shall at last be answered.

"When he opened the fifth seal, I saw underneath the altar the souls of them that had been slain for the word of God, and for the testimony which they held: and they cried with a great voice, saying, How long, O Master, the holy and true, dost thou not judge and avenge our blood on them that dwell on the earth?" (Rev. 6.9–10) During their days on earth these souls had followed the footsteps of the Lamb, their Master. They had no political ambition nor had they exerted any political influence. Now, though, their prayer is directed towards the coming of the kingdom.

(2) *The position of Christians.* Christians should not organize a political party, nor should they exercise political power. Whatever the Lord participated in, in that we can do and participate in, too. As He was, so are we. Such is the position of us Christians. The Lord Jesus said, "My kingdom is not of this world: if my kingdom were of this world, then would my servants fight" (John 18.36). This proves that He had not come to set up any political power on earth. In Colossians 1.13 we read that God, "who delivered us out of the power of darkness, . . . translated us into the kingdom of the Son of his love." So we enter another kingdom, even the kingdom of the beloved Son of God. The kingdom we belong to is spiritual, not political, in nature. Neither, too, is it religious in character.

"Our citizenship is in heaven; whence also we wait for a Saviour, the Lord Jesus Christ" (Phil. 3.20). On what ground do Christians stand? We stand firmly on the ground that we are citizens of heaven. In the days of the Roman Empire, there were two kinds of people: one was the Roman citizens, the other was the Roman subordinates. Those who were citizens possessed public rights. Among other things they could elect and be elected. They enjoyed all the privileges of nation and empire. Those who were subordinates, however, had no public rights. So is it with us Christian believers. Our citizenship is in heaven, and it is *there* that we enjoy our rights. But on earth we are "strangers and pilgrims" (1 Peter 2.11 AV). Though we are indeed given public rights by those nations wherein we dwell, we nonetheless are not eager to exercise these rights. The only right we do exercise is to be law-abiding people. But beyond that, we are not willing to be political persons. All who believe in the Lord are as aliens in the countries where they are born or live.

It is important to note that this kingdom of God has people but no territory, has commands but no law, has love but no armaments. The Lord said, "Go ye therefore, and make disciples of all the nations" (Matt. 28.19a). This would indicate that we do not belong to this earth. Our primary position is heavenly. Today the children of God live on this earth just as Moses did when he sojourned in the land of Midian or just as the children of Israel did when they stayed for a time in Egypt: we, like these before us, try our best to please our neighbors and to help them. During these two thousand years God's children were never to be occupied with the things of this world, to vote, or to delight in touching the realm of secular politics. An Englishman once said that he had been a believer for sixty years and that he knew nothing about casting a vote. He stood outside of any earthly kingdom.

If we truly understand this principle and live in the spiritual, heavenly kingdom, we shall come to recognize that all the political activities of the Roman Church are wrong. During the time of the ministry of the apostle Paul there were believers in many places. So numerous were the Christians in Rome, for example, that tens of thousands had to be killed to get rid of them. Yet the apostle did not exploit the multitude of believers to organize them into a kind of political party, nor did he ever use any or all of the Christian assemblies to obtain or assert political power. When Claudius Lysias, the chief captain of the Roman legion stationed at Jerusalem, questioned Paul, he asked, "Art thou not then the Egyptian, who before these days stirred up to sedition and led out into the wilderness the four thousand men of the Assassins?" (Act 21.38) Men cannot but think that with so many people imbibing his teaching, there must be at Paul's command some political power. But Paul never lifted a single finger to exploit such a situation to any political advantage. Yet the Roman Church has often manipulated the mass of her adherents as a basis for exerting political strength. Today we need to recover the position that Paul took— which is, to stand totally outside of all politics.

(3) *Unwillingness to govern other people.* Christians have only one aim, which is, to maintain a spiritual life, to maintain the grace of God in this age. In accordance with the command of our Lord, the Christian reaction is to be one of grace and not justice. One must turn

the other cheek when his right cheek is smitten. Yet if that be the case, how, then, could one ever be a political ruler? A person can never be a ruler if he lives, acts and reacts under the principle of grace and not under the principle of justice. But in maintaining justice he would fail to be a Christian, that is to say, he would fail to react as a Christian should. Hence the follower of Christ cannot be a ruler, whether great or small in jurisdiction.

Nevertheless, Christians do recognize the political authority set up by God. We cannot subscribe to anarchy. We believe that if anyone sheds blood, his blood should also be shed (see Gen. 9.6). We believe in the death sentence. And therefore God must establish government to implement this. Yet we as Christians cannot act in the role of executioner. This does not mean, however, that such must be the case with those of the world. No; but even so, the left cheek, the inner cloak, the second mile—these reactions taught by our Lord in His so-called Sermon on the Mount—must be kept and observed by Christians; whereas an eye for an eye, a tooth for a tooth, a hand for a hand, a foot for a foot (see Ex. 21.24, Deut. 19.21; see also Matt. 5.38)— these are still the reactions followed by the world. Christians, however, should be different, though we do believe that the soul that sins must die. Few are those who are ready to stand on the kingdom ground of the Sermon on the Mount.

We believe in government and should support the government. Yet we are a peculiar people, willing to suffer. We do not *preach* suffering; we preach the gospel. Yet we are *willing* to suffer if called upon by our Lord

This is our own position. Let us exhort new believers that during this period while our Lord is in heaven we must be willing to suffer.

"Already are ye filled, already ye are become rich, ye have come to reign without us: yea and I would that ye did reign, that we also might reign with you. For, I think, God hath set forth us the apostles last of all, as men doomed to death: for we are made a spectacle unto the world, both to angels and men" (1 Cor. 4.8-9). Believers are to be listed as the last of all, as men doomed to death. For a believer to rule as a king on earth today is out of order. It is true that, in the Old Testament time, people such as Joseph, Daniel, Mordecai, and Esther were rulers. Yet these never aspired to or sought after the public offices in which they served. Furthermore, they were all captives in foreign countries and had no choice in the matter. Let us not touch the politics of this world, especially its authority to rule. The word of God teaches us Christians how to be good people; it has no word telling us how to be secular rulers.

(4) *What our attitude towards government should be.* We should be in subjection. "Let every soul be in subjection to the higher powers: for there is no power but of God; and the powers that be are ordained of God. Therefore he that resisteth the power, withstandeth the ordinance of God: and they that withstand shall receive to themselves judgment. For rulers are not a terror to the good work, but to the evil. And wouldest thou have no fear of the power? do that which is good, and thou shalt have praise from the same: for he is a minister of God to thee for good. But if thou do that

which is evil, be afraid; for he beareth not the sword in vain: for he is a minister of God, an avenger for wrath to him that doeth evil. Wherefore ye must needs be in subjection, not only because of the wrath, but also for conscience' sake. For for this cause ye pay tribute also; for they are ministers of God's service, attending continually upon this very thing. Render to all their dues: tribute to whom tribute is due; custom to whom custom; fear to whom fear; honor to whom honor" (Rom. 13.1–7).

We who are older in the Lord need to read this passage to new believers. Let us teach them that our path is to be in subjection to the higher powers. This is our ground. We do not exercise authority ourselves; we leave that to the people of the world to exercise such power. We should be those who love to submit ourselves to authorities, for we acknowledge that all powers come from God since He is the One who ordains them. So far as the principle of authority goes, it comes from God and not from men. Even as human affairs are ordered by God, so authorities are ordained of God, too. Therefore, he who resists authority withstands the ordinance of God. How we need to learn to be in subjection to all authorities, whether high or low: we must not resist. As believers let us not ourselves touch political things, but let us be in subjection to those in political power. In this world God has committed authority to people of the world. Hence he who resists the power withstands the ordinance of God, thus bringing upon himself judgment.

In verse 4 Paul says: "he is a minister of God to thee for good . . . [and] he beareth not the sword in vain."

Since authority is set up by God, we must be in subjection to him who wields that authority. For he is to punish the evil and to reward the good. Even if he should punish the good and reward the evil (which has indeed happened in the history of government), this frequent phenomenon merely falsifies the divine injunction of punishing the evil and rewarding the good but it cannot change the principle.

In verse 5 we read: "ye must needs be in subjection, not only because of the wrath, but also for conscience' sake." Punishment comes from man, but conscience comes from God. The failure to be in subjection will not only bring on punishment but an uneasy conscience as well. In verse 6 we see that the government God sets forth on earth calls for revenue to maintain its expenses. To pay tribute is also to be in subjection. Whatever statutes the govenment proclaims as law concerning material things, we need to be in subjection to them.

In verse 7 the attitude we Christians should have is summarized: "Render to all their dues: tribute to whom tribute is due; custom to whom custom; fear to whom fear; honor to whom honor." This is a fundamental command of God. Let Christians keep this attitude.

(5) *Our subjection — it has its limits.* Does this mean that we must obey *whatever* is commanded by earthly authorities? No, our subjection is limited. To all authorities who are lower than God himself, our obedience is *relative.* God alone is the object of our *absolute* obedience. Sometimes government orders appear to be unlimited. Whenever these orders are in conflict with God's commands, however, we cannot give unlim-

ited subjection to them. Pharaoh decreed that all the male children born to the Israelite families must be killed. But a midwife and Moses' mother kept the child alive. And in the New Testament Book of Hebrews, this act was commended by God as being of faith. For they were obeying the command of God. Daniel's three friends refused to worship the golden image that Nebuchadnezzar had set up. They disobeyed the order of the king in order to please God. Although their action was serious in its consequences even to the point of death, they would not compromise their faith. King Darius signed an interdict forbidding anyone to ask a petition of any god or man for thirty days except of him. Daniel knew that the ruling of the king had been signed, but he went into his house, with the windows in his chamber opened towards Jerusalem, kneeled down and prayed to God as he had done previously. For this act of disobedience he was cast into the den of lions, but God shut the lions' mouths. Here Daniel was ready to sacrifice his very life, for he could do nothing else (see Ex. 1.17, Heb. 11.23, Dan. 3.17–18 and 6.10).

In Matthew 2.13–14 we learn that Herod sought to destroy the baby Jesus by commanding the slaughter of all the male children in Bethlehem two years old and under; Joseph, however, took the child and fled to Egypt. In Acts 5.29 we find that when the high priest had charged the apostles not to teach in the name of the Lord Jesus, Peter and the apostles answered and said, "We must obey God rather than men."

"Let every soul be in subjection to the higher powers" (Rom. 13.1). In Greek, there are two words for "subjection." One means "obedience," and the other means "submission." The first is a matter of action, the second bespeaks the matter of attitude. What is employed here in Romans is the word for attitude, but what Peter used in his answer to the high priest is the word for action. It is not right to obey men rather than God. We must give absolute submission to all higher authorities. To them our submission is absolute, but our obedience is something relative.* If your father asks you to do something against God's will, you cannot obey in doing it, yet you must still maintain a submissive attitude.

(6) *Initiate no revolution for ourselves.* Our submission has no limit, but our obedience has its limit. To God, we render absolute submission and absolute obedience; to men, our obedience is relative, though our submission can be absolute. When any earthly government illegitimately touches on matters of our Christian faith, we still give them unlimited submission, though we have to disobey; yet we will not start a revolution for our own sakes. Because we are Christians we will not be revolutionaries. Apart from matters of faith, we are able to hear and follow. Today we who are not of this world preach the gospel to save sinners and to satisfy their spiritual needs. On the other hand, men

---

*For a more thorough discussion by the author of this important distinction between *obedience* to authority and *submission* to authority, see "The Measure of Obeying Authority," which is Ch. 11, Part One of Watchman Nee, *Spiritual Authority* (New York: Christian Fellowship Publishers, 1972), pp. 107–12.—*Translator*

on earth do have physical and psychological demands: but let these be fulfilled by the people of this world.

(7) *Concerning the matter of war.* The Bible shows us that God is a Warrior. The wars fought in Canaan were ordained by God. Therefore we cannot say that war is altogether wrong. However, today we are on this earth as messengers of peace. Our Lord did not fight while He was on earth. He declared, "My kingdom is not of this world: if my kingdom were of this world, then would my servants fight" (John 18.36a). Jesus also said to Peter, "Put up the sword into the sheath" (John 18.11a). He does not call us to fight. For all the purposes of God are for peace. All the swords of Christians must remain in their sheaths.

Some may object and argue, "Did not the Lord say, 'let him sell his cloak, and buy a sword'?" (Luke 22.36) In that instance our Lord was asking His disciples if they had lacked anything when He had sent them forth without purse, wallet or shoes at the time of their going out two by two to preach (see Luke 10.1,4; cf. also Matt. 10.5, 9–10 and Mark 6.7–9). This was the time of our Lord's being manifested on the earth, and the disciples had been sent forth as His emissaries to the House of Israel. Then He continued by saying, "But now, he that hath a purse, let him take it, and likewise a wallet; and he that hath none, let him sell his cloak, and buy a sword." This was because He was now to be crucified between two robbers—which meant that He was now being rejected. Formerly He and His disciples had for the most part been received and welcomed; but today He was to be rejected and therefore the time had changed. But the disciples did not understand what they heard. They immediately replied, "Lord, behold, here are two swords." And the Lord said to them, "It is enough" (see Luke 22.35–38). This meant that He was disappointed at their not understanding what He had said. They interpreted the Lord's use of the term sword literally, whereas He had used it metaphorically. What He meant by it was that the time had changed: they could no longer expect welcome and hospitality; on the contrary, from now on they must learn to take care of themselves in this hostile world. That He did *not* mean a *literal* sword is proven by the fact that shortly afterwards when Peter used a sword, the Lord explicitly told him to put the sword back into its sheath (see John 18.10–11).

Do we Christians oppose war? We ourselves will not fight, for we stand on Christian ground; yet we do not oppose war, for this is a matter that belongs to government. Governments may engage in war. But we Christians must keep the teaching of Christ.

During the war between France and Prussia (1870–71), one servant of the Lord wrote in substance as follows: If Christians become soldiers and fight, they have become fallen Christians. No one can choose to fight in this matter of war. Fighting for the sake of patriotism can only be reckoned as having spiritually fallen. If some feel compelled to do so, we have nothing to say. It is a matter between them and the Lord. But the Spirit of God in this age is love and is peace-loving. If a Christian brother is drafted he should say to the authorities that he believes souls are eternal. And that thus, if the person on the other side is a brother, he (the would-be draftee) cannot fight against him. And if he (who is on the other side) is a sinner, he cannot fight against him either, lest he send a soul to the eternal lake of fire. So Christians should not be soldiers and fight wars.

With this that the servant of the Lord has written long ago we would agree.

6 | Waiting for the Coming of the Lord*

Ye come behind in no gift; waiting for the revelation of our Lord Jesus Christ. (1 Cor. 1.7)

They themselves report concerning us what manner of entering in we had unto you; and how ye turned unto God from idols, to serve a living and true God, and to wait for his Son from heaven, whom he raised from the dead, even Jesus, who delivereth us from the wrath to come. (1 Thess. 1.9,10)

Our citizenship is in heaven; whence also we wait for a Saviour, the Lord Jesus Christ. (Phil. 3.20)

The grace of God hath appeared, bringing salvation to all men, instructing us, to the intent that, denying ungodliness and worldly lusts, we should live soberly and righteously and godly in this present world; looking for the blessed hope and appearing of the glory of the great God and our Saviour Jesus Christ. (Titus 2.11-13)

---

*Again, the readers of Watchman Nee, as was said in a footnote about the previous chapter's message, may notice some similarities

According to the teaching of the Bible, the Lord Jesus Christ not only has died for me for my justification and risen and ascended to be my High Priest to intercede for me and to manage my affairs as the Mediator, but He also will come again to this earth. Let us look into this matter of His coming again more closely.

(1) There are many passages in the Scriptures which explicitly tell us of the second coming of the Lord. He himself has said, "I go to prepare a place for you ... I come again, and will receive you unto myself; that where I am, there ye may be also" (John 14.2c–3). In Acts 1.10–11 we are told that as the Lord was ascending to heaven, two men in white apparel appeared and said, "Ye men of Galilee, why stand ye looking into heaven? this Jesus, who was received up from you into heaven, shall so come in like manner as ye beheld him going into heaven." Hebrews 9.28 declares: "Christ also, having been once offered to bear the sins of many, shall appear a second time, apart from sin, to them that wait for him, unto salvation." Apart from sin, at His second coming. Revelation 22.20 says: "He who testifieth these

---

between the message now translated and published here for the first time and another message entitled, in this case, "The Second Coming of the Lord" which appears on pages 67–78 of Watchman Nee, *The Spirit of Judgment* (New York: Christian Fellowship Publishers, 1984). This latter message, like the contents of the preceding chapter of that book, was one of the Basic Lessons the author had presented at Mount Kuling in 1948. But it must be repeated here that a year later at the 1949 Session the author had a different purpose in mind which accounts for whatever differences exist between the two messages.—*Translator*

things saith, Yea: I come quickly. Amen: come, Lord Jesus." By that time, all of the twelve apostles had died except John. The holy city Jerusalem had been sacked and destroyed. The Holy Spirit had already come. The Lord himself had come and returned to heaven. Yet He still testifies that He is coming quickly. From all these passages, therefore, we can be assured that there is not just the first coming of Jesus but there is also to be His second coming.

Each Lord's Day the Church gathers to remember the Lord until He comes (see 1 Cor. 11.26). Such remembrance will not cease until He returns in glory. Each remembrance causes us to wait for His coming. Yes, He does not come only once, He comes twice. This second coming of His is as factual as the event of His cross. At His coming the second time all the problems and the history of sin will be resolved. The cross is where sin was judged; the second coming is when sin will be concluded. We are given so many testimonies surrounding the second coming of the Lord.

(2) What kind of attitude can be deemed to be truly reflective of a waiting for the Lord? Let it be clear at the outset that it is not a waiting for the *teaching* of His coming: it is a waiting for Him himself. Let us carefully read the Scripture passages quoted above to new believers so that they may enter into a right understanding of what it means to wait for the Son of God to come from heaven. Suppose you have a master who says that he will come to you on July 1st. Will you just sit there and do nothing? Or will you set out to prepare for his coming? The proper attitude is waiting.

It is a mistake merely to study prophecies out of curiosity. That is not the right way to wait.

What, then, is waiting? It is doing all things with an eye that looks for the Lord's coming. Whatever He commands we perform. Thus we behave as those who are waiting for Him. We wait for Him as servants wait for their master. During the time of waiting we will not beat our fellow-servants but will be faithfully serving Him (see Luke 12.40–46). This may be a long wait. For He only tells us that He may come at any time. Indeed, there are signs that need to be fulfilled. We find that there are five major signs: (a) that which concerns the Jews, (b) that which concerns the Roman Church, (c) that which concerns the Church, (d) that which concerns the world, and (e) that which pertains to general conditions.

(3) Concerning the sign of the Jews, in 1948 the nation of Israel came into being. After nearly two thousand six hundred years had passed, that nation has once again been revived. Because of this, God's children should come into an awareness of the soon coming of the Lord. We ought to assume an attitude of waiting daily. Let us show new believers that believing in the Lord's second coming and studying it is one thing, while waiting for His coming is another far different thing. There are not many who are of the latter type. Upon believing in the Lord your attitude should undergo a drastic change, just as is told of in 1 Thessalonians 1.9–10: that a person "turn unto God from idols ... to wait for his Son from heaven." To study prophecies such as those relating to the Millennium and so forth

is something extra. Your attitude must experience a significant change, otherwise your all will still be focused on earth. As you believe in the Lord you become a heavenly, new creation waiting for the coming of the Lord. You are not as those who *write* about the second coming, but as people who *wait* for the Lord's coming. You are a citizen of heaven, an anointed one. To wait for the Lord's coming is the goal of your life. Everything is changed, because you have touched "the city which hath the foundations, whose builder and maker is God" (Heb. 11.10). You pin no hope on anything on this earth. Your all is laid on this waiting for the second coming of the Lord.

Of all people in my entire life, Miss Margaret E. Barber has left me with the deepest impression of all. She truly was one who waited for the Lord's coming. In her mind and heart it would be an *un*expected thing if the Lord did *not* come. Once I spent the end of an old year with her. On New Year's Eve she prayed, "Lord, if You will, You can still come tonight. You do not need to wait till next year." Her face was set towards the coming of the Lord. Do we know that our purpose for being here on earth is not a waiting to serve the Church but a waiting for the Lord's coming? If we believers are not careful we can easily allow some other thing to become a substitute for the coming of the Lord. If so, this would be a fall.

On one occasion Miss Barber had written a poem about the second coming of the Lord. There was one word in the poem I did not understand. It was the word "corner." She therefore said she would show the meaning of it to me. Whereupon she immediately walked to a corner, and as she went around the corner she said she might meet the Lord. How our Lord is waiting every day to come. The time of His coming is drawing nearer and nearer. And it might be that it shall be at a corner where He will be seen first. Here was a person who truly was waiting for the Lord's coming. Her whole life was engaged in preparation and waiting for this very event. Day after day she lived to await the coming the Lord.

In what way does our Lord's second coming differ from His first coming? What will He do at His second coming that is different from His first? We know that at Jesus' first coming He came to deliver people from sins and to give them access to God and a new power by which to live. This, however, is but half of salvation. To be free from sin and to possess a liberated life leaves the very presence of sin undealt with. It is true that with the Lord's first coming we become liberated people, people who are set free from the power of sin; nevertheless, sin is still present in this world. Hence, salvation remains incomplete. One might, for example, fall into the hands of bandits and later get freed from their power, but the bandits may not yet have been destroyed. Just so, in His second coming, our Lord shall come to destroy, as it were, "the bandits" so that sin no longer will be present. The cross at Jesus' first coming gives us inner freedom; His second coming brings in deliverance in environment. The first time brings in the saving of the life; the second time brings in the saving of the whole man.

In His first coming, therefore, the Lord Jesus deals with life; in His second coming, He will deal with environment. Today we have new life; at His second coming we will have a new environment to supplement this new life.

With the Lord's first coming, our body can still die; with His second coming, this transformed body will be undying. After His first coming, this body of ours is still left fragile, thus limiting the work of God. After His second coming, however, this body will be redeemed and be free from all weaknesses and limitations. Christians at the first coming may enjoy inner victory, but living in Sodom is nonetheless painful. Sin is our near and ever present neighbor. The more we are delivered from the power of sin, the more we sense the presence and sinfulness of sin. How we long for the second coming of the Lord, for then we will be saved environmentally as well as physically: no more death, no longer any weakness, and no more thorns.

People under persecution particularly look for the coming of the Lord. So is it for those who hate sins. How wicked the world around us is. But at His second coming, not only the problems of sin and death will be resolved, even Satan and all his powers — "the bandits," if you will — shall be destroyed. Under grace we are able to perceive that the whole world lies in the hands of the evil one. Though his power is great, the first coming of the Lord enables us to overcome the enemy's power. The second coming takes us further on, for our Lord will dissolve Satan's power and solve all the problems of sin in the environment and death in the body. This should cause us to be filled with unspeakable joy and praise!

We must wait for the Lord's second coming for Him to implement the completion of His finished work.

Some people cannot understand why the Church preaches the gospel of personal salvation and not a gospel for the society. We do believe in a social gospel a well as a personal gospel, but we recognize that there is a time for each. At His second coming, the social gospel will be preached and implemented. Today the Lord has not called us in His Church to be preoccupied with social and political concerns (other than with what Christ himself was involved when healing the sick and feeding the poor and needy). But the world is very much preoccupied with such concerns, and greatly utilizes science, for example, to support society. Instead, we in His Church today cause society to touch life. What *we* do is that which the world *cannot* do. We help people in society to obtain salvation. But at the second coming of the Lord, the external as well as the internal will both be saved. In His first coming, Jesus saves souls. In His second coming, He will save society as well. Today we do primarily a spiritual work and let others deal with the great social problems confronting the world.

(4) Many fundamental problems of the world will be solved. Let us touch upon each of these briefly. (a) *The problem of injustice and the Lord's second coming.* Today there are those who oppress and those who are oppressed. There are those who deprive and those who are deprived. There is injustice in material things as well as injustice in the psychological realm. Sometimes people are so pressed and oppressed that they rise up in revolt, but they in turn soon begin to oppress others. In Isaiah 11.4 the Lord is recorded as saying: "with righteousness shall he judge the poor, and decide

with equity for the meek of the earth; and he shall smite the earth with the rod of his mouth; and with the breath of his lips shall he slay the wicked."

(b) *The world's great problem of war.* In the entire recorded history of the world, in but 268 years of it has there not been war! Wars can be divided into two kinds: civil and international. Since the First and Second World Wars, the nations have been preparing for a coming Third World War. War comes from human lusts. In Isaiah 2.4 the Lord declares, "He will judge between the nations, and will decide concerning many peoples; and they shall beat their swords into plowshares, and their spears into pruning-hooks; nation shall not lift up sword against nation, neither shall they learn war any more." They will not learn war anymore. This is social salvation indeed!

(c) *Diseases that fill the world.* Science invents many medicines. But as medicines increase, so do the number of diseases. For example, many bacteria increase their resistance after being treated with sulfa drugs. They cannot be killed. After a few days the sickness will return and must be treated again. According to the records of Leviticus and Deuteronomy in the Old Testament, sin and disease are closely related. Sickness or disease is at times a judgment upon sin. But at the second coming of the Lord, this problem will be completely resolved. For we read in God's word that in the new heaven and new earth "the leaves of the tree [the tree of life] were for the healing of the nations" (Rev. 22.2; see also Eze. 47.12).

(d) *The problem of famine will be solved.* Due to man's sin the earth has been cursed (see Gen. 3.17ff.)

and does not yield the total fruit it at one time could have. That which is useless grows profusely, but that which is useful does not grow or grows in less quantity. Famine today is a general phenomenon. Even the application of fertilizers does not guarantee a rich harvest. But all will be resolved at the second coming of the Lord. It is prohesied in Isaiah 49.8–10: "Thus saith Jehovah, In an acceptable time have I answered thee, and in a day of salvation have I helped thee; and I will preserve thee, and give thee for a covenant of the people, to raise up the land, to make them inherit the desolate heritages; saying to them that are bound, Go forth; to them that are in darkness, Show yourselves. They shall feed in the ways, and on all bare heights shall be their pasture. They shall not hunger nor thirst; neither shall the heat nor sun smite them: for he that hath mercy on them will lead them, even by springs of water will he guide them." Indeed, there shall be rivers in the desert, and the earth will not yield up weeds anymore. Moreover, all strifes among men related to the obtaining of food will totally cease.

(e) *The problem of education.* Some people are educated, some others are not. But at the coming of the Lord they shall not teach every man his neighbor, for as Hebrews 8.11 says: "they shall not teach every man his fellow-citizen, and every man his brother, saying, Know the Lord: for all shall know me, from the least to the greatest of them."

(f) *The problem of places of sin.* Today this world is full of places of sin, such as taverns, opium dens, cinemas, dancing halls, and so forth. These places provide convenience for people to sin. There are more opportunities for sinning provided in cities for the more affluent people. But when the Lord shall come, "the Son of man shall send forth his angels, and they shall gather out of his kingdom all things that cause stumbling, and them that do iniquity" (Matt. 13.41). All these instruments and places of sin will be eradicated.

(g) *The problem of animal cruelty.* Today a portion of the living creatures are in a state of pain and suffering. Both the higher and the lower animals are being cruelly treated. Domesticated animals as well as wild animals are all subject to atrocious treatment at the hands of man. There can be no peace between men and a tiger. There is hardly any place for a lion anymore in this so-called civilized world. Human beings ill treat all kinds of animals. No wonder all the animals groan and travail in pain, waiting for deliverance (see Rom. 8.19–22). At the coming of the Lord, though, these sighings will come to an end: "the wolf shall dwell with the lamb, and the leopard shall lie down with the kid; and the calf and the young lion and the fatling together; and a little child shall lead them. And the cow and the bear shall feed; their young ones shall lie down together; and the lion shall eat straw like the ox. And the sucking child shall play on the hole of the asp, and the weaned child shall put his hand on the adder's den. They shall not hurt nor destroy in all my holy mountain: for the earth shall be full of the knowledge of Jehovah, as the waters cover the sea" (Is. 11.6–9). What a great deliverance, what a glorious liberation!

(h) *The problem of political powers shall be solved.* Over the centuries men have used political power to oppress people. One day all the kingdoms of the world shall become the kingdom of our Lord and of His Christ, as is spoken of in Revelation 11.15. There will be no more political oppression. The earth shall be filled with righteousness and peace. Without the salvation that comes with the second coming, salvation is not complete. Day by day our faith in the coming of the Lord is strengthened and increased. For we are confident that at His coming all these problems shall be resolved.

What, then, should be our attitude in this world? We know that many in the world are not saved. Their primary need is life. The winning of souls to the Lord is the responsibility of us believers. We must preach the gospel to get them saved. We are entrusted by the Lord with this primary work of the Church. Of course, we also help them the best we can as fellowmen — especially the sick, the poor and the needy. At His first coming our Lord came for sinners who live in a sinful world. We who now are saved are righteous people living in a sinners' world. But at His second coming we shall be a righteous people dwelling in an environment of righteousness — that is to say, living in a righteous world. For this reason, let us exhort new believers that apart from fulfilling their human duties they are to win lost souls for Christ who is their only hope. All the other problems will be fully resolved at the second coming of the Lord. The signs in this world tell us that His coming is near.

7 | Martyrdom

Fear not the things which thou art about to suffer: behold, the devil is about to cast some of you into prison, that ye may be tried; and ye shall have tribulation ten days. Be thou faithful unto death, and I will give thee the crown of life. (Rev. 2.10)

I know where thou dwellest, even where Satan's throne is; and thou holdest fast my name and didst not deny my faith, even in the days of Antipas my witness, my faithful one, who was killed among you, where Satan dwelleth. (Rev. 2.13)

The local church of Smyrna suffered greatly. If they would be faithful unto death, they were promised the crown of life. Martyrdom is the way to the crown. "Ye shall have tribulation ten days" (Rev. 2.10). This indicates a not very long period. This local church stands for the Church after the apostolic age, that is to say, during the second and third centuries after Christ.

In the letter to the church at Pergamum the Lord says: "I know where thou dwellest, even where Satan's throne is; and thou holdest fast my name, and didst not deny my faith, even in the days of Antipas my witness, my faithful one, who was killed among you, where Satan dwelleth" (Rev. 2.13). In the preceding letter, the letter to the church at Smyrna, the Lord had declared: "the devil is about to cast some of you into prison" (2.10). Here at Pergamum it is more than a matter of persecution or tribulation; it is a matter of being killed, which is martyrdom. All these are the works of Satan.

According to the letter to the church at Pergamum it would seem as though in persecuting this local church, Satan had established a definite location for his throne there. Though he roams over the earth as a roaring lion, seeking whom he may devour, just as it has been described in the Book of Job and in one of Peter's letters, he also has his specific earthly dwelling place. He sets his throne there to facilitate his work of persecuting the saints or killing God's children. It may be in Pergamum, Rome, Lyon or London that he sets up his throne to carry out his nefarious works. Nevertheless, the Lord exhorts us, "Be thou faithful unto death" (2.10).

He calls us to be martyrs for Him. Under whatever circumstances, even being persecuted to the point of having our life threatened or taken, we are encouraged to be faithful unto death. We are to give up our lives. The Lord's demand is nothing less than life itself.

When Antipas, of the church at Pergamum, was killed, there was at least one in Pergamum who was faithful unto death. How amazing it is that for these two thousand years no ones knows who this Antipas was. Even though the Church throughout the entire world does not know him, the Lord does, and pays particular attention to him. How great is the attention of the Lord towards those who are killed for His name's sake. "Anti" means "greatest" or "in opposition to"; "pas" means "all people." In other words, when all people are against the Lord, he is willing to stand with the Lord against all. Martyrs are acknowledged by the Lord as being faithful.

Let us tell this to new believers. Let them see that all who believe in the Lord Jesus should be willing to lay down their lives for Him. Believers are expected to give up their lives for the sake of Christ as well as to believe in Him. It is declared by the Lord Jesus, as recorded in Matthew 10:18: "yea and before governors and kings shall ye be brought for my sake, for a testimony to them and to the Gentiles." It is further declared in verse 21: "brother shall deliver up brother to death, and the father his child: and children shall rise up against parents, and cause them to be put to death." The Lord anticipates hatred by the world towards Christians. The history of the Church during these past two thousand years has been intertwined with the hatred of the world. To accept the Lord is to be hated by the world. Believers will be brought to the place of death, though they may not necessarily die. Nevertheless, they must be prepared to be faithful even to death if necessary. The demand of martyrdom is upon every believer. Said Jesus: "be not afraid of them that kill the body, but are not able to kill the soul: but rather fear him who is able to destroy both soul and body in hell" (Matt. 10.28). Satan can only kill the body, but he cannot kill the soul.

Once when a sister in the Lord was brought before a judge, she was smiling. The judge was so enraged that he ordered her to be beaten. Yet she told the judge, "You may destroy my body, but you cannot kill my soul. I have such inner peace that I cannot help smiling." Let us explain to young believers that many have testified the word they preached with their own blood. Young Christians need to be reminded that people such as Stephen, James, Peter, Andrew, Matthew, Matthias, Bartholomew, Thomas, Paul, Mark, Luke, Barnabas, Timothy and Ananias were all martyrs. They, too, like these martyrs of old, must be faithful unto death.

Yet why is there martyrdom? It is because the world is against Christ. They hate Him without a cause: "ye shall be hated of all men for my name's sake," once said the Lord; "but he that endureth to the end, the same shall be saved" (Matt. 10.22). It is Satan who instills such hate in men, and he is the one who stands behind their backs.

One historian has written about the Christian martyrdom which had occurred during the first two centuries after Christ. He stated that except for the day of January 1, no less than five thousand believers had been killed every day! One can therefore say that in those days the gospel was preached with blood. The blood of the martyrs was indeed the seed of the gospel and of the Church. All this happened because Satan hates the name of Christ. That which the world does is evil, so they who are of the world shun the light (see John 3.19,20). Believers, however, are faithful to the Lord and confess His name before men. "Every one therefore who shall confess me before men," the Lord promised, "him will I also confess before my Father who is in heaven" (Matt. 10.32).

Christian martyrdom is different from the rest of martyrdom in that Christian martyrs are those who are able to flee but do not flee, whereas other martyrs are people who cannot escape. Some Christians were forcibly brought before idols and given incense to offer to those idols. At their refusal to do so, these believers were thrown to be eaten by wild beasts. They could have saved their own lives by renouncing the Lordship of Christ and offering to idols, but they refused to deny their Lord. Furthermore, at the time of the Roman persecutions, if anyone would confess Caesar as god, he would be released; but if he would not confess Caesar as god, he would be killed. Let all children of God know that they must confess the name of the Lord under any circumstances. The world at best can only kill the body; it cannot kill the soul. Therefore, let us not be afraid of the world.

During the martyrdom of these Early Church believers many of them exhibited such courage and serenity that the spectators were deeply moved. Indeed, there are stories of Roman soldiers who, after they had killed Christians, themselves believed in the Lord Jesus and asked to be killed. "I hold not my life of any account as dear unto myself, so that I may accomplish my course, and the ministry which I received from the Lord Jesus, to testify the gospel of the grace of God" (Acts

20.24). So declared Paul. And such is the way of the Church. After the deliberations of the council in Jerusalem recorded in Acts 15, James and the other apostles and elders wrote a letter to the brethren who were of the Gentiles in Antioch, Syria and Cilicia, in which they described Barnabas and Paul as "men that have hazarded their lives for the name of our Lord Jesus Christ" (v.26).

Let us now note the ways which lead to martyrdom. There are basically two: (1) persecution from the secular world; or (2) persecution from the religious world. We find in John 16.2 these solemn words of our Lord Jesus: "They shall put you out of the synagogues: yea, the hour cometh, that whosoever killeth you shall think that he offereth service unto God." In Revelation 13 we read of the Antichrist, the man of sin, who will "make war with the saints, and ... overcome them" (v.7). In Revelation 17 the woman mentioned therein, and variously called there the Great Harlot, Mystery, Babylon the Great, the Mother of Harlots and of the Abominations of the Earth, is seen "drunken with the blood of the saints, and with the blood of the martyrs of Jesus" (v.6). Such have been the ways of persecution and martyrdom during these past two thousand years.

As we have learned, during the first two hundred years after Christ, tens of thousands of believers were martyred at the hands of the Romans throughout the Roman Empire.

[*Translator's Note:* The author then narrated several stories of persecution and martyrdom of brave believers at the hands of the Romans, culled from such sources as John Foxe's *Book of Martyrs* and Eusebius's *Ecclesiastical History.*]

But the persecutions and martyrdoms the believers in the Church have suffered during the centuries thereafter have come mostly at the hands of the Roman Catholic Church, and these persecutions were most severe.*

[*Translator's Note:* Again, the author then narrated several more stories of believers having bravely faced terrible persecution and martyrdom, this time at the hands of the Roman Catholic Authorities; these tragic incidents were also derived from Foxe's *Book of Martyrs* and other sources.]

The way of the Christians has never been interrupted, despite the terrible circumstances many have endured for the sake of Christ. During the past two thousand years, these children of God have all had faith. And their reward shall be that they shall reign with Christ in the coming kingdom: "I saw thrones, and they sat upon them, and judgment was given unto them: and I saw the souls of them that had been beheaded for the testimony of Jesus, and for the word of God, and

---

*However, it also needs to be pointed out, as the author would readily agree, that segments of the Protestant Church have not been guiltless in this regard either. The tragic persecution of the dissenter Michael Servetus in Geneva by the followers of John Calvin is but one, albeit extreme, example that quickly comes to mind. In 1553 he was burned at the stake, crying aloud through the flames: "O Jesus, thou Son of the eternal God, have pity on me." Quoted in Kenneth S. Latourette, *A History of Christianity* (New York: Harper & Brothers, 1953), p. 759.—*Translator*

such as worshipped not the beast, neither his image, and received not the mark upon their forehead and upon their hand; and they lived, and reigned with Christ a thousand years" (Rev. 20.4).

Notice that on each throne there is someone sitting. Four things are mentioned; namely, (1) the overcomers will have the power of judgment; (2) some are the souls of them who had been beheaded for the testimony of Jesus; (3) some are the souls of them who had been beheaded for the word of God (pointing to the Old Testament saints); and (4) some are those who had not worshiped the beast nor received the mark of the beast, who are the martyrs of the Great Tribulation. These four classes of people shall reign with Christ and receive the kingdom. They shall receive the crown of life, which is a sign of authority. For this cause they willingly and gladly put themselves in the hand of the Lord. Their tribulations are great, but their exceedingly great glory is far greater: "Every one therefore who shall confess me before men, him will I also confess before my Father who is in heaven" (Matt. 10.32)—"I will confess his name before my Father, and before his angels" (Rev. 3.5). The overcomers are those who confess the name of the Lord Jesus before men. They will in turn be confessed before the Father and the angels by the Lord. This is to say that they shall reign with Him in the kingdom.

We are told in God's word that in the last days "brother shall deliver up brother to death, and the father his child: and children shall rise up against parents, and cause them to be put to death" (Matt. 10.21). No time is as serious as the present.* Let us tell new believers that all these martyrs have with one accord confessed that the Lord has shown special grace to them.

---

*It should be noted that even as the author was speaking at the Second Workers Training Session in the Mount Kuling area located just outside Foochow in southern China (and held continuously throughout the spring and summer of 1949), the Chinese civil war was fiercely raging very nearby between Nationalist troops and the ultimately triumphant Communist forces of Mao Tse-tung. — *Translator*

8 | Idol Worship*

And there came one of the seven angels that had the seven bowls, and spake with me, saying, Come hither, I will show thee the judgment of the great harlot that sitteth upon many waters; with whom the kings of the earth committed fornication, and they that dwell in the earth were made drunken with the wine of her fornication. And he carried me away in the Spirit into a wilderness: and I saw a woman sitting upon a scarlet-colored beast, full of names of blasphemy, having seven heads and tens horns. And the woman was arrayed in purple and scarlet, and

---

*This message by the author should not in any sense be construed by the reader as an attack on the communicants personally who are within the Roman Catholic Church. It is, however, to borrow a phrase from Paul the apostle of the Lord, a "speaking of the truth in love" where there has been a departure from Biblical truth as a consequence of Roman Catholic teaching and practice. In that sense, the message has been included in the present volume as a warning to new believers against whatever is not of God.

Additionally, the reader will notice that on several occasions

decked with gold and precious stone and pearls, having
in her hand a golden cup full of abominations, even the
unclean things of her fornication, and upon her forehead
a name written, MYSTERY, BABYLON THE GREAT, THE
MOTHER OF THE HARLOTS AND OF THE ABOMINA-
TIONS OF THE EARTH. (Rev. 17.1–5)

Today we will discuss the matter of idol worship.
Revelation 17.4 states: "the woman was arrayed in purple and scarlet, and decked with gold and precious stone
and pearls, having in her hand a golden cup full of
abominations, even the unclean things of her fornication." This woman points to the Church system of
Roman Catholicism.** As with the woman here por-
trayed in Revelation 17, so Romanism is full of gold,

---

the author is found quoting statements and passages from an
unnamed source but which he has described as "a well-known
and approved book of the Roman Church." Unfortunately, this
particular reference volume, apparently written by a member of
the Roman Catholic Church and apparently approved by it, could
not—after an extensive search—be located by the translator. The
latter has therefore been forced in most instances to translate
directly from the author's text regardless whether or not the results in English constitute exact quotations of such statements
or passages as have been derived by the author from that work.
—*Translator*

** The reader should consult the pertinent portion, "Babylon and
Her Destruction (17.1–20.6)," of Watchman Nee's commentary
on the complete book of Revelation entitled *"Come, Lord Jesus"*
(New York: Christian Fellowship Publishers, 1976), pp. 178–216
especially pp. 178–189, wherein the author thoroughly discusses
the reasons for why he believes this woman points to religious
Rome, i.e., the Roman Catholic religious system.—*Translator*

silver and precious stones and is also resplendent with purple and scarlet. The Catholic pope wears two crowns: one is ecclesiastical, the other is political. These are made of gold, with 146 large precious stones and 540 pearls. The golden cup full of abominations signifies idolatry, as the following passages of Scripture will affirm.

"The graven images of their gods shall ye burn with fire: thou shalt not covet the silver or the gold that is on them, nor take it unto thee, lest thou be snared therein; for it is an *abomination* to Jehovah thy God. And thou shalt not bring an *abomination* into thy house, and become a devoted thing like unto it: thou shalt utterly detest it, and thou shalt utterly abhor it; for it is a devoted thing" (Deut. 7.25–26). "He shall make a firm covenant with many for one week: and in the midst of the week he shall cause the sacrifice and the oblation to cease; and upon the wing of *abominations* shall come one that maketh desolate; and even unto the full end, and that determined, shall wrath be poured our upon the desolate" (Dan. 9.27). "He [Manasseh] did that which was evil in the sight of Jehovah, after the *abominations* of the nations whom Jehovah cast out before the children of Israel" (2 Chron. 33.2). "I said unto them, Cast ye away every man the *abominations* of his eyes, and defile not yourselves with the idols of Egypt; I am Jehovah your God. But they rebelled against me, and would not hearken unto me; they did not every man cast away the *abominations* of their eyes, neither did they forsake the idols of Egypt. Then I said I would pour out my wrath upon them, to accomplish my anger against them in the midst of the land of

Egypt" (Eze. 20.7–8). In all these passages, abominations refer to idols.

The points to notice are: (1) the woman holds in her hand, and uses, "a golden cup full of abominations" (idols) and other "unclean things of her fornication"; and (2) she gives, to the point of drunkenness, this cup of abominations to the people who dwell on the earth—which means, therefore, that she spreads idolatry to the entire world (see both Rev. 17.4 and 17.2, respectively). Now of all the idols they worship, that of Mary tops the list. Because there was no goddess in early Christianity, the Roman Church specially created such a goddess. They picked out Mary to be worshiped. From the *veneration* of Mary, it gradually developed into the *worship* of Mary. She is considered to be holy. Many things have been said about Mary.

In a well-known and approved book of the Roman Church, these words of different Catholics are recorded: None can be saved without Mary. The way of salvation is opened through her. Why hesitate and not pray to her? The holy God of glory calls us to seek for grace; but without the intercession of Mary no one could receive grace. Whoever prays for grace without the intercession of Mary is like one who tries to fly without wings. When people asked Pharaoh for food, he sent them to Joseph. Today Christians can say to Mary that their salvation is in her hand. Raymond Jordan (?) said, "Our salvation is in Mary's hand." Another has said, "All who are saved must depend absolutely on the favor and protection of Mary. All who are so favored and protected by her are saved; otherwise they will perish instead of being saved."

Thus does the Roman Church join salvation and Mary together. Now look at the relationship of Mary to the Lord. The same book cited above continues by saying that Mary is eternally grateful to the Son for having chosen her to be His mother. Neither can it be denied that the Son is grateful to Mary, because she gave the human nature to Him. As a recompense to her, Mary receives special honor and all her requests will be answered.

In the third chapter of this book approved by the Roman Church, and in that chapter's first section, it is written that as the Scriptures record that just as for the sake of love the Father gave us His Son to die for us, so also did Mary. Whenever she permits, she gives us His Son. There is also in this section of Chapter Three of the book a story about a bird being taught to say "Hail, Mary." When a big bird came to catch it, it chirped "Hail, Mary," and the big bird fell down and died. And the interpretation given in the book is that even as an ignorant bird is answered by calling on Mary, so much more shall a person who calls upon her be delivered. The book went on to indicate that all who hold offices in the Holy Church should raise their voices to chant "Hail, Mary" or to declare that she is the hope of sinners.

A Catholic canonized saint once declared that the blessed Virgin can do whatever she pleases in heaven or on earth. Then addressing Mary directly, this same Catholic saint said the following: All the powers in heaven and on earth have been given to you. There is nothing you cannot do. You can cause all the disappointed to receive salvation. The Lord has already exalted you. Whatever He can do, you can also do, for this is His good pleasure.

One Catholic has said: Mary, your protection is almighty. Another answered: Indeed, Mary is almighty; her authority extends throughout the earth and transcends the law of any nation. Whatever the authority of the Son is, so is the authority of the Mother. An almighty Son, an almighty Mother.

Someone else declared: God has not only put the whole Church in the grace of Mary, He has also placed it under her authority.

In the record of the holy chronicle, there is discussed a parable of two ladders. The Lord stands at the top of the red ladder, while the holy Mother stands at the top of the white ladder. Many who climb the red ladder tumble down. Hence they are told to climb the white ladder. It is easy to climb up, for the holy Mother stretches out her hand to help them to get to heaven.

Is not such a parable as the above ridiculous?

A Catholic, Dennis (?) by name, has said: Who are the saved? Who are the people who will reign in heaven? They are those for whom the compassionate Mother has interceded. Mary says (quoting from Proverbs): "By me kings reign, and princes decree justice" (8.15). Through my intercession, she adds, souls may reign as well as control their lusts. Dennis went on to say that in the future all who reign in heaven will confess that it is Mary in heaven who permits them to enter into heaven according to her will and command.

Such is the glory of Mary in the eyes of Catholic writers.

Heaven and earth and light were created through

the word of God. This is made clear in the Bible. But Catholic teaching propounds the idea that in like manner God became Man such as we are through the command of Mary. Catholic teaching propounds further that the virgin became what it calls "the Mother of God." Therefore, the Catholic Church reasons, she must be exalted to the level of the Godhead. Moreover, no one can be saved without the help of Mary; in the thinking of this Church God has ordained that He will give no grace except through the hand of Mary.

How deep is the fall of Roman teaching! We must show new believers what Mary herself announced: "My soul doth magnify the Lord, and my spirit hath rejoiced in God my Saviour" (Luke 1.46–47). Mary needed the Savior just as we do. It is only through the Lord Jesus that anyone can come to God. The Catholic teaching puts Mary in the place of the Son as the one through whom men come to the Father. The very nature of the gospel has been confused. Our Lord said, "I am the way" (John 14.6a). He also declared: "I am the door" (John 10.9a). He is the One who sits on the throne of grace. If Mary is brought in, the Lord has to abdicate His own throne. This truly is heresy. The center of heresy is with Mary.

Once a friend of D. M. Panton visited Rome and saw many people worshiping Mary. If the Lord manages salvation, but Mary is easier to approach and ask, then she takes away the Lord's position. The fact is that only the Lord is our Savior before God. How many are the idols worshiped in the Roman Church! People have worshiped the statue of Mary, the statue of God the Father. There is an image of the Son, there are images of the twelve apostles and of many canonized saints. To be canonized two requirements must have been fulfilled: a person must (1) have performed miracles, and (2) have lived a holy and pious life. In Catholic teaching saints such as these not only have satisfied God's demand, they also have more virtues in surplus. Accordingly, they have the authority to dispense their extra virtues to us. It is really surprising how people could believe in such a thing. The famed Catholic theologian of the thirteenth century, Thomas Aquinas, wrote in his work the following thoughts: These saints have additional virtues left over and stored up. They are so compassionate that they allow the Church to dispense these accumulated virtues at will. These virtues are sinless, therefore a portion of them may be taken out to meet the need of your sin, thus delivering you from that particular sin.

Such a theory by Thomas shows a total ignorance of the Lord, for is there any sin too great for the Lord to forgive that the saints must be invoked? What grace is there that people cannot obtain from the Lord, so that they must needs seek the help of Mary? Truly the golden cup of religious Rome is full of idolatrous abominations.

[*Translator's Note:* The author here makes a digression of several lengthy paragraphs dealing with the inquisition and other unbiblical past practices indulged in by Roman Catholic authorities that are not germane to the central issue of idol worship under discussion.]

The Roman Empire will be revived; and along with

it, religious Rome will flourish in even greater measure than she has in the past. We need to read to young believers the word in Revelation 18.4: "I heard another voice from heaven, saying, Come forth, my people, out of her,* that ye have no fellowship with her sins, and that ye receive not of her plagues." We would warn all the children of God to keep themselves from the Roman Catholic Church system. We should be alert to its teachings and its practices especially with regard to the worship of Mary and other idols in its midst. May the Lord deliver us from such entanglement.

----

*For a thorough discussion of how the word "her" is interpreted by the author as referring to religious Rome (i.e., Roman Catholicism) as well as political Rome, see again Watchman Nee, *"Come, Lord Jesus"*, pp. 201–5, especially p. 201f. The reader should note particularly page 202, where the author writes: "'Come forth, my people, out of her'—This is a command. Although it is given at this juncture [Rev. 18.4], it certainly is applicable to those in view in Chapter 17 as well, because there are true believers in the Lord even in religious Rome."—*Translator*

9 | The Judaizers

I know thy tribulation, and thy poverty (but thou art rich), and the blasphemy of them that say they are Jews, and they are not, but are a synagogue of Satan. (Rev. 2.9)

Behold, I give of the synagogue of Satan, of them that say they are Jews, and they are not, but do lie; behold, I will make them to come and worship before thy feet, and to know that I have loved thee. (Rev. 3.9)

In both the letter to the church at Smyrna and the letter to the church at Philadelphia, our Lord shows us how the Jews disturbed both churches. How seriously has Christianity been tampered with by Judaism. A slight carelessness will bring in Judaism. The priests of the Old Testament become our pastors today. Law regulates our behavior. Festivals are made mandatory of us. All this began at Smyrna and was practiced in Philadelphia. In the nineteenth century a group of people in the Church rose up and overcame the Judaizers.

But up to the present, there yet remain the works of the Judaizers in the Church. The Protestant Church succeeded the Roman Church, but neither have their communicants been freed from the bondage of Judaism either. Let us therefore spend time to show new believers how to deal with this influence. In this message today we will deal with the Judaizers in the Church from the perspective of their attitude towards the law.

Of the Ten Commandments, the fourth one concerns the Sabbath day, which is Saturday. It is a mistake, say certain Judaizers, to observe it on the Lord's Day. Let us see if this notion is in accordance with the teaching of the Scriptures, as is claimed by its adherents.

First of all, what do the Scriptures teach about the law? God never gave it to the Gentiles. He gave it to the nation of Israel: "He showeth his word unto Jacob, his statutes and his ordinances unto Israel. He hath not dealt so with any nation: and as for his ordinances, they have not known them. Praise ye Jehovah" (Ps. 147.19–20). It is the explicit teaching of the Bible that the Gentiles do not have the law: "When Gentiles that have not the law do by nature the things of the law, these, not having the law, are the law unto themselves" (Rom. 2.14).

(1) How about the Gentiles after they are saved? Acts 15.5 reads: "there rose up certain of the sect of the Pharisees who believed, saying, It is needful to circumcise them, and to charge them to keep the law of Moses." Nevertheless, the decision of the council at Jerusalem was: "it seemed good to the Holy Spirit, and to us, to lay upon you [Gentile believers] no greater

burden than these necessary things; that ye abstain from things sacrificed to idols, and from blood, and from things strangled, and from fornication; from which if ye keep yourselves, it shall be well with you" (Acts 15.28–29). The Gentiles do not have the law *before* they are saved, and they are not required to keep the law *after* they are saved. For God has not given the law to the Gentiles.

(2) How about the Jews? The law was given to the Jews. They are born under the law. "Till heaven and earth pass away, one jot or one tittle shall in no wise pass away from the law, till all things be accomplished" (Matt. 5.18). The Lord has no intention of destroying the law among the Jews, for they are under the law. "To fulfil" (5.17) means to fill it to the full. For example, formerly it was: "Thou shalt not kill"; today, says Jesus, it is: Thou shalt not hate. This is to fill the law to the full.

(3) Many Jews have believed in the Lord. How about their relationship to the law? When the Jews become Christians, they belong to the Church in which there is neither Jew nor Gentile (see Col. 3.11). Paul illustrates it this way: "are ye ignorant, brethren (for I speak to men who know the law), that the law hath dominion over a man for so long time as he liveth? For the woman that hath a husband is bound by law to the husband while he liveth; but if the husband die, she is discharged from the law of the husband. So then if, while the husband liveth, she be joined to another man, she shall be called an adulteress: but if the husband die, she is

free from the law, so that she is no adulteress, though she be joined to another man. Wherefore, my brethren, ye also were made dead to the law through the body of Christ; that ye should be joined to another, even to him who was raised from the dead, that we might bring forth fruit unto God" (Rom. 7.1-4).

For a Jew to believe in the Lord is like a woman getting married. How can she be freed from the former husband, the law? There is only one way—if the husband dies. But here is a problem: As we have read already, heaven and earth may pass away, but one jot or one tittle of the law shall not pass away till all things be accomplished. What can be done if the law never dies? Well, even if the *law* does not die, *you* can die. How? "Ye also were made dead to the law through the body of Christ." So the teaching of Romans 7.1-4 is that though the law cannot die, God has caused us to die with Christ, and thus we are freed from the law. Through the death of Christ we are set free from the law. We are raised from the dead with Christ and then married to Him. This death is real death. Hence, in being joined to Christ, we are no adulteress. God uses the death of Christ to include our death. How assured this is. And resurrection is also sure.

Hence, a man (even a Jew) who has formerly been under the law has died and been raised in Christ to receive new life. He is not under law anymore since he has already died. "Sin shall not have dominion over you: for ye are not under law, but under grace" (Rom. 6.14). Furthermore, "now we have been discharged from the law, having died to that wherein we were held; so that we serve in newness of the spirit, and not in oldness of the letter" (Rom. 7.6). In believing in the Lord, one is discharged from the law. The position of a Christian is that he has died. It is a position of death, he having been crucified with Christ. The law has no relationship with him, it having only a relationship with the old man.

(4) We must show new believers why God gave the law. There is a good reason for it, made clear in the Scriptures. "Now this I say: A covenant confirmed beforehand by God, the law, which came four hundred and thirty years after, doth not disannul, so as to make the promise of none effect. ... What then is the law? It was added because of transgressions, till the seed should come to whom the promise hath been made; and it was ordained through angels by the hand of a mediator. ... Is the law then against the promises of God? God forbid: for if there had been a law given which could make alive, verily righteousness would have been of the law. ... But now that faith is come, we are no longer under a tutor" (Gal. 3.17,19,21,25).

These words explain why the law was given and how we are delivered from the law. Four hundred and thirty years before God gave the law He had already promised to Abraham that "in thee shall all the families of the earth be blessed" (Gen. 12.3b). Abraham believed God and was thus reckoned to be righteous. His descendants also shall be saved through faith, for the promise of God is according to the gospel of grace. Before the gospel of grace is accomplished, there is first the promise. Yet to receive grace, there must also be transgressions. For if men have no need, they cannot accept grace. Yet in the sight of God all are sinners. But men themselves do not know that they are sinners. They need to sin before they know themselves to be sinners. How can they know they have sinned? By giving them the law. With the coming of the law comes also a knowledge of trangression. For example, there has been coveting, but to man it is not known to be sin. But after God says, "Thou shalt not covet" (Ex. 20.17a), coveting trangresses the law, thus becoming sin. The use of the law is to expose to man the sin of man. "Thou shalt not make unto thee a graven image . . .; thou shalt not bow down thyself unto them, nor serve them" (Ex. 20.4a–5a). Man's making a hundred golden calves as images is not known to be sin, not till the law was proclaimed by God to the people from the heavens (see Ex. 20.1–6, 20–23).

Abraham was reckoned by God as righteous because of his faith. This too was the covenant of the Lord, the Abrahamic Covenant. Yet, as Paul has said, how untrustworthy were men. Accordingly, four hundred and thirty years after that covenant was made, God gave men the law. The law was to be kept, and yet it did not disannul the covenant God had made with Abraham and his descendants. Then what is the use of the law? "What then is the law? It was added because of transgressions, till the seed should come to whom the promise hath been made" (Gal. 3.19). With the law added, there comes transgression. Thus God is able to put His covenant into effect. Sin was originally present, but the sinner could not receive the grace of God because he had no knowledge of his sin. Now, though, he has sinned against the law; and so, he is able to receive grace.

The law will continue on till the Lord Jesus shall come. "For all the prophets and the law prophesied until John" (Matt 11.13). The function of the law is to fulfill the promise. The end is grace, and the means is law. The law must be used to bring people into grace.

Do law and grace oppose each other? No. Wrote the apostle Paul: "before faith came, we were kept in ward under the law, shut up unto the faith which should afterwards be revealed. So that the law is become our tutor to bring us unto Christ, that we might be justified by faith" (Gal. 3.23–24). The law is God's servant, leading us to Christ. Once we touch Christ, we are no longer under the tutor anymore, that is, under the law. Hereafter we do not live under law, nor do we follow it any longer. For the more we keep the law, the more hopeless we are. Nevertheless, it has led us to Christ. The law, therefore, is not to be considered a hindrance.

(5) Some argue that even though we are saved by Christ and not by the law, we still need to keep the law after we are saved. Let us again look into the Letter to the Galatians and discover how it deals with such people. The apostle Paul maintains that as it was useless for man to keep the law for justification, so it is equally needless for man to keep the law after being justified through faith in Christ. Some Judaizers had urged the Galatian believers to keep the law. "I marvel," said the apostle Paul, "that ye are so quickly removing from him that called you in the grace of Christ unto a different gospel; which is not another gospel: only there are some that trouble you, and would pervert the gospel of Christ" (Gal. 1.6–7). If you were not able to keep the

law before, you are still unable to keep it now. Paul went further by saying, "If any man preacheth unto you any gospel other than that which ye received, let him be anathema" (v.9). "Anathema" means "accursed."

"If I build up again those things which I destroyed, I prove myself a transgressor" (2.18). Whoever is to preach a gospel of another kind is to be cursed. If I build up this other and false gospel, I am a transgressor. For Christ has died to the law so that I might live unto Him. "I have been crucified with Christ; and it is no longer I that live, but Christ liveth in me" (v.20a). Only one who is living can again be put under the law. Since I have died with Christ, who will possibly be put under the law save Christ who lives in me? It is absolutely impossible. So I who now live unto Christ can never again be put under the law. The law speaks to the natural man; it cannot speak to the man who is dead.

"O foolish Galatians, who did bewitch you, before whose eyes Jesus Christ was openly set forth crucified? ... Are ye so foolish? having begun in the Spirit, are ye now perfected in the flesh?" (3.1,3) The law has its demand upon the flesh, but you are in the Spirit. It would be going backward if you try to be perfected by keeping the law.

"The fruit of the Spirit is love, joy peace, long-suffering, kindness, goodness, faithfulness, meekness, self-control; against such there is no law" (5.22–23). "Against such there is no law" may also be interpreted as "against which there is no control of the law." For the fruit of the Spirit is not under the control of the law. That which violates the law is the flesh; that which keeps the law is also the flesh. The fruit of the Spirit is beyond the reach of the law. If you try to keep the law, it is your flesh that attempts it. As the law enters in, the Holy Spirit ceases to be active. The moment you think of keeping the law, immediately the flesh comes forth. It is far better if you do not try to keep the law, for the object of the law is the flesh. So this is Christianity.

Since the law cannot give us justification, how can we who have been justified in Christ return again to the law? If we are not careful, we may easily be Judaized. People who do not understand God's plan and arrangement of salvation always attach themselves to the law. When God gave the law to men, His purpose was not for them to keep the law for the law's sake. It did not say that keeping the law would satisfy His heart. The reason for asking them to keep the law was to obtain the righteousness according to the law. To not covet, to honor father and mother, and to not worship idols—all these are reckoned as righteousness. So the keeping of the law is not for the sake of honoring the law, but rather for the purpose of attaining to the righteousness according to the law.

Here we have (i) the keeping of the law, (ii) the righteousness according to the law, and (iii) the receiving of life before God. The righteousness according to the law comes through the keeping of the law, but who is able to keep the law? Now through Christ we have received life. After we have received life the Judaizers would tell us we must still keep the law. Yet this is recalling the old man back to life. We are saved because God has put us into the death of Christ. We are reckoned righteous through the blood of our Lord. In Him we receive a new life which is not subject to the keeping of the law. In order to again keep the law the flesh must be revived to keep it. For this new life has no need of keeping the law. When we receive life, the righteous requirement of the law is already fulfilled in us. There is no need for us to keep it. "That the ordinance [mgn: "requirement"] of the law might be fulfilled in us, who walk not after the flesh, but after the Spirit" (Rom. 8.4). "Do not covet" is the law. "Not coveting" is righteousness. We today refrain from coveting because of the righteousness which comes from the life of Christ. We do not need to keep the law, and yet we have the righteous requirement of the law. This is the gospel. Christians do not covet—yet this does not come from the law that says: "Do not covet"; it comes from the righteousness of the Holy Spirit. This truly is the gospel!

The law does not end in itself. It ends in righteousness. But now apart from the law, God has used another means to produce righteousness. We are not justified by keeping the law; therefore, once being justified we have no obligation to keep the law. Now because life does not come from keeping the law, so it is useless for us to keep the law after we have been saved and received new life. We have been crucified with Christ. We are not justified by keeping the law. The righteousness of God comes to us through faith in the finished work of Christ on the cross. Having begun in the Holy Spirit, we now must be perfected in the same Spirit. It is the Holy Spirit who works in us that righteousness.

"But now that ye have come to know God, or rather to be known by God, how turn ye back again to the weak and beggarly rudiments, whereunto ye desire to be in bondage over again?" (Gal. 4.9) "For freedom did Christ set us free: stand fast therefore, and be not entangled again in a yoke of bondage" (5.1). "Wherefore, my brethren, ye also were made dead to the law through the body of Christ; that ye should be joined to another, even to him who was raised from the dead, that we might bring forth fruit unto God" (Rom. 7.4). Everyone who has received life is joined to Christ. Through the death of Christ a Christian is raised from the dead that he might be joined to Christ. He not merely receives life; he actually is joined to the life of Christ. So a saved person is one who has been raised from the dead and is joined to Christ. He is married to Him. Whoever tempts him to go back to law makes him an adulteress. This is to be accursed.

In the latter part of Romans 7.4 it says: "that ye should be joined to another, even to him who was raised from the dead, that we might bring forth fruit unto God." It does not say, do not worship idols. It says that we bear or bring forth the fruit of the Holy Spirit, and one of the fruits is not worshiping idols. We are not to produce the righteousness according to the law by keeping the law, but to fulfill the righteousness of the law through the fruit of the Holy Spirit. There is the righteousness of the law without the need of keeping the law.

Now concerning the keeping of the Sabbath, we have seen in the days of the local church at Smyrna that the Judaizers came in. Later, during the ascendancy of the Roman Church, Judaism and Christianity became deeply intertwined. For over a thousand years the Lord's

Day was called the Christian Sabbath. Furthermore, a century ago the Judaizers came into the Church again and commanded people to keep the Sabbath. They even hung the text of the Ten Commandments in church buildings. They considered the Sabbath, which is Saturday, to be the Lord's Day. Yet Saturday is the Sabbath of the Jews, while Sunday is the Lord's Day of the Christians. The Christians do not keep the Sabbath day of the Fourth Commandment. It is highly improper to change the Sabbath, which is the seventh day of the Jewish week, to the first day of the week. The real issue, however, does not lie in which day of the week it is. It rests in the fact that Christians do not keep the Sabbath, for we believers are not under the law.

Let us see what the Scriptures teach about the Sabbath: (1) The first mention of it is found in Genesis 2.3: "God blessed the seventh day, and hallowed it; because that in it he rested from all his work which God had created and made." From that time, for the next two thousand five hundred years nothing further was heard about the Sabbath. (2) After leading the children of Israel out of Egypt, God gave the Sabbath to them in the wilderness: "See, for that Jehovah hath given you the sabbath, therefore he giveth you on the sixth day the bread of two days; abide ye every man in his place, let no man go out of his place on the seventh day" (Ex. 16.29). (3) The Sabbath became law: "Remember the sabbath day, to keep it holy. Six days shalt thou labor, and do all thy work; but the seventh day is a sabbath unto Jehovah thy God: in it thou shalt not do any work, thou, nor thy son, nor thy daughter, thy man-servant, nor thy maid-servant, nor thy cattle, nor thy stranger that is within thy gates: for in six days Jehovah made heaven and earth, the sea, and all that in them is, and rested the seventh day: wherefore Jehovah blessed the sabbath day, and hallowed it" (Ex. 20.8–11). (4) You as the people of God must keep My Sabbath day for this is a sign between you and Me throughout the generations. So instructs the word of God in the Old Testament: "Speak thou also unto the children of Israel, saying, Verily ye shall keep my sabbaths: for it is a sign between me and you throughout your generations; that ye may know that I am Jehovah who sanctifieth you. ... It is a sign between me and the children of Israel for ever: for in six days Jehovah made heaven and earth, and on the seventh day he rested, and was refreshed" (Ex. 31.13,17)—"Moreover also I gave them my sabbaths, to be a sign between me and them, that they might know that I am Jehovah that sanctifieth them" (Eze. 20.12). (5) To keep the Sabbath is the salvation of the Jews. It is quite evident that the Sabbath is given to the Jews as a sign.

What does Paul teach concerning the Sabbath? He maintains that the Sabbath is a thing that has passed away: "having blotted out the bond written in ordinances that was against us, which was contrary to us: and he hath taken it out of the way, nailing it to the cross ... Let no man therefore judge you in meat, or in drink, or in respect of a feast day or a new moon or a sabbath day: which are a shadow of the things to come; but the body is Christ's" (Col. 2.14,16–17). "The bond written in ordinances" refers to the entire law. On the cross our Lord has blotted out the entire law. This is because the law attacks us and demands us to be holy.

But we are sinful. So the Lord was crucified for us. The Judaizers argue that what has been blotted out is the ceremonial law, but that the moral law was not taken away. Feast days, new moons and Sabbath days are not classified by them as being under ceremonial law. Therefore, they must be kept, even as the moral law under the Ten Commandments.

However, the Scriptures do not make such a distinction. All the ceremonial laws are for moral purposes. To offer sacrifice is for a moral reason. Colossians shows us that what has been blotted out is not merely the ceremonial law. "The bond written in ordinances" refers to the total contract God made with Israel. It is the same as when we sign a contract today. In Exodus 19.5 we read: "Now therefore, if ye will obey my voice indeed, and keep my covenant, then ye shall be mine own possession from among all peoples: for all the earth is mine." And in verse 8: "all the people answered together, and said, All that Jehovah hath spoken we will do." There is the bond written in ordinances. It refers to moral and not only to ceremonial law. So let us cause new believers to see that for us Christians it has already been nailed to the cross.

In Romans 7.7 we see the presence of the law: "What shall we say then? Is the law sin? God forbid. Howbeit, I had not known sin, except through the law: for I had not known coveting, except the law had said, Thou shalt not covet." But in Colossians 2.14 we see that the law has been taken out of the way, having been nailed to the cross. Verse 16 follows verse 14. Because the law has been taken out of the way, therefore meat or drink or feast day or new moon or sabbath day have all passed away. According to Exodus 19.8, there is no reason to divide the law into ceremonial and moral law. Christians therefore are not subject to these laws.

The Judaizers immediately retort that the Sabbath day mentioned in Colossians 2.16 is not a regular Sabbath day. It is the Sabbath day of a feast. But the Greek original shows the number to be plural here: "sabbaths." It therefore includes the Sabbath days of the weeks as well as the Sabbath days of the feasts; otherwise, why should the Sabbath be mentioned after citing the feast, which already includes its Sabbath day? Accordingly, no one has the authority to say that the Sabbath day of the week is excluded from the meaning of Colossians 2.16.

Furthermore, the Judaizers in Colosse were not as interested in the Sabbath days of the feasts as they were concerned with the Sabbath days of the weeks. That is why Paul wrote the letter to the Colossians in order to show them that all these things had passed away. Only in modern days have people tried to separate the Sabbath days of the weeks from the Sabbath days of the feasts.

In the same verse (2.16) the apostle declares, "Let no man therefore judge you ... " In other words, these things are not worthy to be judged; for these things are "a shadow of the things to come; but the body is Christ's" (v.17).

"Wherefore, my brethren, ye also were made dead to the law through the body of Christ; that ye should be joined to another, even to him who was raised from the dead, that we might bring forth fruit unto God" (Rom. 7.4). As Christians we have been discharged from the law of the former husband. The Judaizers, however, debate the point and remonstrate that the law here refers only to ceremonial law. How absurd is their reasoning. In verse 7 Paul notes this: "I had not known coveting, except the law had said, Thou shalt not covet." This is one of the Ten Commandments. It is moral, not ceremonial. So "if the husband die, she is discharged from the law of the husband" (Rom. 7.2b). "The law of the husband" is the law of the Ten Commandments.

"For if the ministration of condemnation hath glory, much rather doth the ministration of righteousness exceed in glory. ... For if that which passeth away was with glory, much more that which remaineth is in glory. ... And [we] are not as Moses, who put a veil upon his face, that the children of Israel should not look stedfastly on the end of that which was passing away ... But if the ministration of death, written, and engraven on stones, came with glory, so that the children of Israel could not look stedfastly upon the face of Moses for the glory of his face; which glory was passing away: how shall not rather the ministration of the spirit be with glory?" (2 Cor. 3.9,11,13,7–8)

Here we see the difference between the ministration of the law and the ministration of the Spirit, the difference between the ministry of Moses and the ministry of Christ. The law condemns, brings in death, and is passing away. This distinctively points to the law written and engraved on stones. The Judaizers again use their sole argument, they saying that the law that ministers death refers to ceremonial law. But we all know that what were inscribed on the stones (the stone tablets of the Ten Commandments) were moral laws.

Today the law of the Spirit is written upon our hearts. In verse 3 we only see the contrast between the tables of stone and hearts of flesh. Thus have we been absolutely freed from the law. God has made Christ our righteousness through the Holy Spirit. There is no need for us to keep the law. Therefore the question of the Sabbath is a thing of the past.

"One man esteemeth one day above another: another esteemeth every day alike. Let each man be fully assured in his own mind. He that regardeth the day, regardeth it unto the Lord; and he that eateth, eateth unto the Lord, for he giveth God thanks; and he that eateth not, unto the Lord he eateth not, and giveth God thanks" (Rom. 14.5–6). Here, two matters are being dealt with: (a) keeping or not keeping a day, and (b) eating or not eating meat. Some people eat vegetables and not meat. Paul says that this person is one who is weak in faith. Likewise, there are people whose conscience bothers them if they do not keep a day. These, again, are weak in faith (see v.1).

In the Old Testament time, a person who did not keep the Sabbath day was to be stoned to death. In the New Testament time, the Jews wanted to kill the Lord for His not keeping the Sabbath. They were not able to carry out their plan because miracles through Jesus were definitely being performed. In the days of Paul, the apostle maintained that "every day [was] alike." Here must have been a change in dispensation. The Sabbath day is a shadow of things to come. There is in the law a portion which serves as type. In the Old Testament, commands to keep the Sabbath day are frequently given. Even in the millennial kingdom the Jews will still offer sacrifices. Yet in the New Testament writings of Paul he did not exhort people to keep the Sabbath day, *not even once.* It would really be strange if the Sabbath day was to be kept and yet was not mentioned *at all.* Thus we realize that the dispensation has changed.

According to Acts 15.22, at the council in Jerusalem the apostles and elders were all present. If the Sabbath day was important, surely it would have been taken up and decided on by the council. But this was not addressed. For the law and the prophets prophesied until John. Christ is now the sum of the law. Hence in the New Testament there is no command that we need to keep the Sabbath day. In Colossians we are told that the Sabbath day has passed away. Paul also maintained—in Romans 14—that to keep or esteem a day or not is something optional.

Finally, nothing in the New Covenant needs to be completed with the help of the Old Covenant. The Roman Church teaches that keeping the Lord's Day is keeping the Sabbath day of Christianity. Yet this is to blend together Judaism and Christianity. Here come the Judaizers who try to bring the entire system of Judaism into Christianity. Yet if we must keep the Sabbath day, then we are no longer Christians. By accepting the Jewish system, we drop the status of being Christians and turn into pure Jews—even as the apostle Paul declared: "Ye observe days, and months, and seasons, and years. I am afraid of you, lest by any means I have bestowed labor upon you in vain" (Gal. 4.10–11).

The Book of Acts is a continuation of the history of Christ as presented in the Gospels. Yet Acts gives facts but no explanations. It is only history and not teaching as well. The completion of the establishment of Christianity came in about 96 A.D. (the date of the writing of the Book of Revelation), that is to say, by the end of the first century. Then was fulfilled what the Lord had predicted: "Howbeit, when he, the Spirit of truth is come, he shall guide you into all the truth" (John 16.13a). All these Jewish influences of which we have been speaking gradually dropped off; Christianity evolved step by step, so that in the Epistles we finally have Christianity in its more complete form. It is important for us to know and to recognize the progress of Christianity. In the Jerusalem council told about in Acts 15 James and the others did not argue over the matter of keeping the Sabbath day. In fact, it never came up. They discussed circumcision. Paul himself had entered the Jerusalem temple to declare the fulfillment of the days of purification. There is nothing surprising for a Jew to be circumcised. However, we hope the brethren today will see the progress and completion of Christian teachings. Then we shall know what Christianity truly and fully is.

When our Lord was on earth He kept the Sabbath day and received circumcision. But the Letter to the Galatians puts an end to this matter of the Sabbath. The same is true with circumcision. Only after 70 A.D. (the Roman destruction of Jerusalem's Temple) could the letters of Paul stand on the pure ground of Christianity. Before that time the Temple and the priests were still present. It was easy to sit on the fence and enjoy both the lamb and the Lamb of God. For this reason we were given the Letter to the Hebrews. The following verse therein points to this changing time: "There remaineth no more a sacrifice for sins" (10.26). Thereafter, people could no longer straddle the fence. Furthermore, Christianity has developed to the point where a word of God resolves all the problems of the past.

If the Jewish Temple existed today we would still have difficulties, for these Judaizers would bring forth such midway things as have been discussed. A fundamental principle to be recognized is that nothing in the Scriptures can be decided midway. These matters of the Sabbath day and the law are both midway things. They cannot be resolved without going to the Epistles. The final word on the teaching concerning the Sabbath is found in Colossians 2.14, which declares: God has "blotted out the bond written in ordinances that was against us, which was contrary to us; and he hath taken it out of the way, nailing it to the cross."

10 | Walk in the Will of God*

The reason why so many believers make no progress in their spiritual life is either because they do not walk in God's will or because they do not know how to walk in God's will. They have in their mind so many thoughts—each seeming to be God's will—that they cannot discern what is the right walk. Due to their not walking according to the will of God, their spiritual lives remain stagnant. To those who do not at all seek after God's will, I would beg them to do so. They must not be independent and follow after their own will, for God is our Redeemer who has the right to have us obey His will. Indeed, this is quite proper, whether the mat-

---

*This message was first delivered in Chinese by the author at a Friends Revival Meeting presumably sometime in 1924, was later revised by him at Nanking on 4 November 1924 in preparation for publication as an article, and subsequently published in Chinese in *Spiritual Light* magazine —a Christian periodical which was then appearing in China. It is here translated and published in English for the first time. — *Translator*

ter be viewed from the perspective of rights or from that of love. His great love has so constrained us that we cannot help but seek to do His will.

For those who do not know how to walk in God's will, I would ask you to pay attention to the following considerations.

(1) We must walk in the *direct* will of God and not in His *permissive* will. The direct will of God is that original mind in the heart of God which He commands us (or guides us) to follow. The permissive will of God, on the other hand, is that which He permits us to do after our (offtimes persistent) entreaties. Let us take the following as an example: The parents see the need one day of an outing for their children. So they take them out for a day. Days later, their children wish to take another trip because they love the beautiful scenery they witnessed the first time. The parents, however, do not see such a need. Yet due to their children's persistent request and their failure to persuade the children otherwise, the parents finally permit them to go out a second time. Here we see that the first outing is the direct will of parents whereas the second outing is their permissive will. Many believers come to God asking—and even insistently so—for permission to do a certain thing, instead of coming to God inquiring if the thing in question is according to His will. This is truly lamentable!

A review of an incident recorded in the Old Testament will help us understand this matter better. In Numbers 22 we learn that the Moabite king, Balak, had sent emissaries to the prophet Balaam inviting him to come and curse the children of Israel. He promised to give the prophet great rewards, which moved the latter's heart (see Jude 11, 2 Peter 2.15). Balaam indeed wanted to go, but having the fear of God in him, he felt he must ask Jehovah first before any decision was made. "And God said unto Balaam, Thou shalt not go with them; thou shalt not curse the people; for they are blessed" (Num. 22.12). This was unquestionably God's *direct* will. Now after receiving this word from the Lord, Balaam ought to have given up any thought of going. But he told the princes of Balak, "Get you into your land; for Jehovah refuseth to give me leave to go with you" (v.13). How *reluctant in sound* is the word "refuse" that comes from the mouth of the prophet. It was as though Balaam had said to them. "It is not because *I* would not wish to go, but because the Lord does not allow me to go." Whereupon Balak sent princes again to Balaam and promised to promote the latter into great honor. So Balaam came to God once more to ask.

How strange, Balaam! Did not God already tell you on your first approach to Him what His mind and will is? Why do you come to ask the Lord again? Do you think because you are moved by great honor that God too will be so moved? Do you think His will is subject to change? Do you not know that He is the same yesterday, today and forever?

Let us clearly understand here that if Balaam had really wanted to do God's will, he should have frankly told these men on their second visit to him: "God already plainly told me last time that I should not go. So, please return. I will never go." But his greediness so overcame him that he came and entreated Jehovah a second time. Then God said to Balaam: "Rise up, go with them" (v.20). What the Lord meant by His words was: "Since I am not able to restrain you, you may simply go." Which thing the prophet did and went his way.

Now many today do not understand why the angel of Jehovah later came to block Balaam's way to kill him, they not realizing that the way of Balaam was crooked before the Lord (see again 2 Peter 2.15,16 and Num. 22.32b). The same is true in the experience of many Christians today in their walk. They know already in their hearts that the Lord does not want them to do certain things, yet they still love to do them. And whenever opportunities come, therefore, they continue to annoy God by asking. Even though they may not do these things for a time, their hearts have nonetheless already departed from God. And if they eventually do get the Lord's permission, who can question the discipline of the Lord which—as in the case of Balaam with the angel of Jehovah—may follow? For this reason, we must get the Lord's "best," not His "second best." Whoever has a heart that is estranged from God and yet seeks the Lord's will as a cover will be disciplined.

(2) We must not take any text of the Scriptures out of context. The will of God has already been clearly declared in His holy word. All who desire to know the will of God need only search the Scriptures and they shall know His mind on a certain matter. Many believers, however, will simply seize upon one or two verses in the Bible as the will of God for them and act accordingly. They do not seek to know how the whole Bible resolves this problem. This is most dangerous.

Please read Matthew 4.7, which states this: "Jesus said unto him [the devil], Again it is written, Thou shalt not make trial of the Lord thy God." "Again it is written." Again! and again! The devil also quoted Scripture in his temptation of Jesus. Had our Lord been like many believers today, He would have thought that He ought to obey the word of the Scriptures which the Tempter had flung at him. Yet did the Lord Jesus obey? Not at all; for He is one who considers the teaching of the *entire* Scriptures. Hence He answered, "Again it is written." For this reason, in our seeking to know the will of God, we must not pluck a text out of context, randomly choosing and accepting a single verse or passage of verses — in isolation — as the teaching of the Scriptures on a specific issue facing us. We always need to search out whatever other Scripture passages might teach on the particular issue or subject confronting us — that is to say, what *further* words may have been written on it. Let us never make a hasty decision. For just as in the past, the devil today often uses an isolated Scripture verse to deceive men, causing them to listen to lopsided doctrines and to practice many things against the word of God, thus violating His will.

Some believers have a strange way of making a decision — they basing it on a text taken out of context. They treat the Bible in the fashion of augury.* When something happens in their life and they find themselves

---

Augury: "divination of omens or portents (as inspection of the flight of birds or the entrails of sacrificial animals) *or of chance phenomena (as the fall of lots)*" (emphasis added). *Webster's Third New International Dictionary of the English Language Unabridged* (1971 ed.), p. 143. — *Translator*

in a quandary, they will place the Bible before them and pray, "O Lord, I am now about to make a decision on a certain matter, but I do not know if this suits Your will. I will open the Bible at random, and whatever verse my eyes first light upon, this I will take as Your direction for me." Or some may say to God: "I shall open the Bible and whatever verse my finger points at, that shall represent for me Your will." Still others will perhaps say this: "I shall now open the Bible, and the verses which I shall see above (or, below) my eye (or, finger), this I shall take as the Lord's direction." Such a manner of seeking the Lord's will is full of error and quite dangerous to pursue. Satan can easily cause your finger to point at the wrong verse or turn to a wrong page. He has many means and opportunities to ensnare us in his plot. When you ought to stay, he moves you to go. When you should speak, he induces you to be silent.

In conclusion, using the Bible as a means of augury is already out of the will of God. It is very difficult and well-nigh impossible to find the Lord's will through a means that is out of His will. We should never seek to know the will of the Lord in this manner. We ought to spend time daily in the Bible so that we come to understand what it plainly teaches on a certain matter. And thus, when such a matter arises, we will not be at a loss and forced to find a Scripture verse as the Lord's will for us.

(3) Let us never do anything if peace is lacking in our hearts: "Let the peace of Christ rule in your hearts" (Col. 3.15a); "Thou wilt keep him in perfect peace,

whose mind is stayed on thee, because he trusteth in thee" (Is. 26.3). When we are confronted with a difficult problem and we do not know how to act in accordance with the will of the Lord, there is a good (though in and of itself not a perfect) way of guidance, which is, to discern if there is peace in our heart. If I do this or that and I have no peace, this shows I should not do it. The word peace here does not simply mean a kind of tranquil feeling. It means that there is an unchanging, proper tranquillity in our spirit. If a thing will cause you to lose the tranquillity of your spirit, it is better for you not to do it. Yet, this is not a perfect means of guidance. Sometimes a thing which ought not to be done gives you peace when you do it and makes you feel unpeaceful if you do not do it. Satan can easily play on our feeling, giving us false peace or false unrest in order to make us do what he wants us to do. Hence, in judging whether or not a matter is God's will, peace is merely a *partial* consideration. We cannot solely depend on it.

(4) Do not look only at environment and need as an indication of God's will. Many in seeking the Lord's will depend on environment as their sole guidance. This will end up in confusion and defeat. Let us look at the story of Jonah. God's will was for His prophet to go to Nineveh, but Jonah decided to go to Tarshish. When he went to the port of Joppa, he indeed found a ship going there. So, he paid the fare and went down into the ship to go to Tarshish (see Jonah 1.3). If the prophet looked solely at environment, he would certainly reckon his escaping from Jehovah as the will of God. Other-

wise, how could there have been such a smooth arrangement? In the first part of verse 3 we read: "Jonah rose up to flee unto Tarshish"; and in the next part of the same verse, it states: "and found a ship going to Tarshish." Not only was there a ship going there, it so happened also that he had money in his pocket to pay for the fare. At this time, therefore, the environment was fully in concord with his thought. If a Christian were to find himself in such a situation today, he too would consider himself to be walking in the will of the Lord. Will he not think as follows?—if I go about seeking the will of God in this way, I shall get the approval of my friends and relatives; thus I do not lose human affections and at the same time I can still serve the Lord. I need not spend lots of money and time, and yet the success will be great. The environment is so perfect that I can proceed or stop as I wish. Do not all these factors show that God is leading me?

Let us go back to the story of Jonah. Did he know that he was out of God's will? Let me tell you, there are plenty of ships going to Tarshish. There is sufficient money to pay for the voyage. Nonetheless, neither ship nor cash can guarantee that your trip to Tarshish is correct. For the will of God is for you to go to Nineveh. Hence, in our seeking the Lord's will, we must not look to environment alone, lest we lose our way.

Furthermore, the greatest attraction in environment is need. We may frequently reflect that because there is need in a certain place and because we are able to supply the lack, that that must indeed be the place to which we should go and render help. Suppose, for instance, that I lack some theological education. And suppose, further, that an opportunity is opened to me to provide this lack. If not careful, I might very well interpret this as God's arrangement for me. To take the element of need in environment as their guidance is the common symptom to be found among the majority of believers when it comes to determining the will of God. Their slogan is: "This needs to be done, so I do it." Let us remember, however, that "needs to be done" may not be what God wants you to do.

Let us look at the example of Paul and his companions: "They went through the region of Phrygia and Galatia, having been forbidden of the Holy Spirit to speak the word in Asia; and when they were come over against Mysia, they assayed to go into Bithynia; and the Spirit of Jesus suffered them not" (Acts 16.6–7). Before the time of verse 6 Paul and his friends had done good works in different places elsewhere. At these places many believers were edified and many sinners were saved. Now they intended to go to Asia (Asia Minor) because the people there seemed to have tremendous needs since many had never heard the gospel that Christ in bearing their sins on the cross had died for sinners such as they. Such great needs among these Asians appeared as though God was leading them to Asia. But no, that was not to be so. The Holy Spirit forbade them to go to Asia. Their thought of going to Bithynia was likely the same, and yet the Spirit of Jesus suffered them not to go there as well. In the light of all this, therefore, it becomes clear that when we seek to know the will of God, we must not depend too much on need that can so easily attract us. For in so doing we may miss the Lord's will.

(5) Do not take the vision or dream as the will of God. Nowadays there are not a few believers in the Church who singularly trust in supernatural phenomena like this as guidance for their actions. They frequently speak of their supernatural experiences, such as when they saw the Lord Jesus and what He said to them; that on a certain night they dreamed of heaven and heard the Lord speak face to face with them regarding what they should do afterwards. Or else that they have had some strange dreams and received such and such interpretations as God's way of directing them to do certain things. Many are the cases like this which can be cited.

Now I do not suggest that all these are false, but I do say that even if these things give us some help we cannot lean on these phenomena alone in knowing the will of God. This is because Satan is quite capable of deceiving believers with false dreams and visions so as to lead them astray from the direct will of God. As a matter of fact I know that many supernatural experiences of many believers are but the disguise of Satan as an angel of light. Not discerning the wiles of the Enemy, God's children end up doing things that do not glorify Him.

We can learn a few things from considering a supernatural experience which the apostle Paul once had. "A vision appeared to Paul in the night: There was a man of Macedonia standing, beseeching him, and saying, Come over into Macedonia, and help us. And when he had seen the vision, straightway we sought to go forth into Macedonia, concluding that God had called us to preach the gospel unto them" (Acts 16.9-10). Now someone may ask, Did not Paul and his fellow-workers decide on the direction of their way by knowing God's will through a vision? The answer is a definite No; for if you read carefully, you will discern that that was just not so. For, first of all, Paul was the only one who saw the vision, yet the decision to go to Macedonia was made by "us." The clear record here is: "*he* [Paul] had seen ... straightway *we* sought to go." Their going to Macedonia was not caused by the vision Paul saw. Yes Paul indeed had a vision, but then he and the others with him were *led of the Lord.* All of them together were of one accord to go to Macedonia. They were not singularly guided by a vision or dream, taking it and it alone as the indication of God's will in the matter. Moreover, the word "concluding" in verse 10 indicates the fact of them all examining the situation before the Lord and deciding together afterwards that God had indeed called them to go and preach the gospel to the Macedonians in Europe.

Hence we see from this that Paul and his companions did not move precipitously merely because of the vision; rather, they weighed the matter very carefully before the Lord in advance of their making the decision to go. In view of this, it ill behooves any of us to rely on these supernatural experiences alone; instead, we should carefully weigh and examine them before the Lord to see if these agree with God's will. Only *then* should any decision be made.

(6) Avoid preconceived ideas lest you fail to receive God's will. One major thing which believers when seeking God's will must avoid is preconception. Having a

preconceived notion about anything prevents us from hearing God's voice. "I verily thought with myself," confessed Paul, "that I ought to do many things contrary to the name of Jesus of Nazareth" (Acts 26.9). Such was the preconceived idea which Paul had had of persecuting the church in his unconverted days when he was known as Saul. He did not know the relationship between Moses and the Lord Jesus. He viewed the latter as a great sinner who had perpetrated a great sin against so-called Judaism. So he determined to wipe out this new religion. He went so far as to give his consent to have believers killed and to force them to blaspheme (see Acts 8.1, 26.10–11). He could do all these unrighteous acts with a good conscience. And why? Because he had thought: "I ought." But he had been wrong. Formerly, he had thought that all he had been doing was according to God's will, not realizing it was the very opposite. His mistake lay in his preconception and private idea. Because he conceived what he formerly did as something "ought," therefore he could not receive God's will.

It is highly natural for us to have preconception and personal opinion about matters or about doing things. We cannot forget the persons who hate us or the things we do not like. We are not willing to seek any solution as to God's will by means of a tranquil and restful heart. We always exalt our preconception and private thought, interpreting these to be God's will. Though we may discover our fault later on, it is already too late. Hence, each time we come to God, we must cast aside all our prejudices and ask the Father to guide us. Even if His guidance is totally contrary to the concept we have held earlier, we should gladly follow Him. Never let us plan and decide first, and then pray, using prayer as a pretence and cover.

(7) Do not be hasty, but wait. Some believers are so used to doing things according to their own idea that it is difficult for them to seek and do God's will in all matters, both big and small. They are like wild horses without a bridle, and are thus uncontrollable. They may sometimes appear to be seeking God's will, but before they get an answer from the Lord they have already taken action. How hasty is our flesh in doing things. It deems seeking and following the Lord's will as too slow. When we seek the Lord for His will, we want Him to tell us right away, so that we may commence doing. No doubt our Lord would gladly tell us His will immediately, but for our benefit—because we are yet unready, or because the time has not come—He cannot show us His mind at once. In such circumstances, we must not be hasty, but rather let us wait patiently upon Him. He will reveal His will to us at the proper time.

How sad that in spite of our desire to seek the Lord's will on a certain matter we do not seek to know how to wait. There is a timing involved. If we seek His will but fail to wait for the time He desires to reveal His will, such seeking is false and the result is nil.

In this very connection, let us look closely at an incident from the Old Testament. "He [Saul] tarried seven days, according to the set time that Samuel had appointed: but Samuel came not to Gilgal; and the people were scattered from him. And Saul said, Bring hither the burnt-offering to me, and the peace-offerings. And he offered the burnt-offering. And it came to pass that, as soon as he had made an end of offering the burnt-offering, behold, Samuel came ... And Saul said, Because I saw the people were scattered from me, ... I forced myself therefore, and offered the burnt-offering. And Samuel said to Saul, Thou hast done foolishly; thou hast not kept the commandment of Jehovah thy God, which he commanded thee: ... but now thy kingdom shall not continue" (1 Sam. 13.8–14a).

Seven days was the time period agreed upon between Samuel and King Saul. Before the seventh day ended, and seeing that Samuel had not arrived, Saul began to offer the burnt-offering. Yet just as he ended the offering, Samuel did come, arriving on time. Saul had rebelled against God's will and was thus reprimanded: and all because he could not wait to the very end. It had appeared to Saul as though Samuel had missed his appointment, so the King began to offer the sacrifice towards the end of the last day. But as soon as he had finished offering, Samuel arrived. Israel's prophet had not broken the agreement; otherwise, how could he have reprimanded King Saul and announced the judgment of God upon him? Saul was denounced because he was too hasty; he could not wait.

Many people act like King Saul. On impulse, they imagine they have to worship God in a certain way, they must arise and do certain work, or they should go to a certain place. So powerful is such inner impulse that they cannot wait but must act straightaway. Do you sometimes feel that a fire is burning within you which drives you to do something at once? You ought to go to sleep, for after a good night's rest, you will find out if such pressure has come from God. Be at rest for a few days. During these few days' quietness God will cause you to understand His will. Let this become a practice in your walk with the Lord. For if such a thought has indeed been injected suddenly in your mind by Satan, it will be calmed down after a good night's sleep or a few days' rest. Let us never act impulsively. Be very sure before any step is taken. Otherwise we too will be reproved by the Lord just as was Saul.

In sum, then, we should wait on the Lord and act only after we have His will. May God protect us from not being able to wait to the last, from not being patient to the end. Let us never "force" ourselves to do anything that we are absolutely certain of, lest we sin against God.

(8) Do not run ahead of the Lord, nor lag behind Him. In this connection, note the following portion of Scripture: "Whenever the cloud was taken up from over the Tent, then after that the children of Israel journeyed: and in the place where the cloud abode, there the children of Israel encamped. At the commandment of Jehovah the children of Israel journeyed, and at the commandment of Jehovah they encamped: as long as the cloud abode upon the tabernacle they remained encamped. And when the cloud tarried upon the tabernacle many days, then the children of Israel kept the charge of Jehovah, and journeyed not. And sometimes the cloud was a few days upon the tabernacle; then according to the commandment of Jehovah they remained encamped, and according to the commandment of

Jehovah they journeyed. And sometimes the cloud was from evening until morning; and when the cloud was taken up in the morning, they journeyed: or if it continued by day and by night, when the cloud was taken up, they journeyed. Whether it were two days, or a month, or a year, that the cloud tarried upon the tabernacle, abiding thereon, the children of Israel remained encamped, and journeyed not; but when it was taken up, they journeyed" (Num. 9.17–22).

Here we see a life — a corporate life at that — which obeyed wholly. Whether the Israelites journeyed or remained in camp depended entirely upon Jehovah. With no regard to place or time — whether it were morning, evening, two days, a month or a year — they only followed the will of the Lord. They neither went ahead nor lagged behind Him. They walked in perfect step with their God.

Yet many believers are not like this. Some walk ahead of the Lord. They have entertained many plans and plots and have now already made up their minds. When they contemplate doing a certain thing, they not only decide on *doing* it, they even know *how* to do it. Then they kneel down and pray: "O Lord, we have planned to do a certain thing. Please help us that we may succeed." Though they confess God as Lord, the fact of the matter is that in essence here is how they pray to God: "Hear, my servant! I now have decided on doing a certain thing, but I cannot do it alone. My servant, come and help me!" How sad that many believers treat their God as a servant and know it not. If we are self-centered, it would be better not to ask for the Lord's help lest we make Him our servant. May we not be so self-centered that we walk ahead and therefore ask the Lord to follow.

Some Christians, however, are just the opposite to these who walk ahead. They instead lag far behind the Lord. In whatever matter which the Lord has commanded, they hesitate to proceed. They view fear and excuse as signs of humility. They never finish the course which the Lord has assigned them each day. Such people act like Moses once did—who made many excuses and greatly hesitated to take up responsibility at the time he was called by God (see Ex. 4.1-17). May the Lord keep us from rushing ahead or lingering behind.

(9) Do not take a prayer answer as the evidence of God's will. Once I asked a Christian, "How do you know this is the will of the Lord?" He said, "Because I have prayed and received an answer." I said, "It is better you do it without prayer." Why? Because what he did was against the Scriptures. Many believers think because they pray and get some sort of response before they act, that what they thereafter do is in conformity to the will of the Lord. This, however, is not so! There is no difference between doing a thing after prayer or doing a thing without prayer *(unless in prayer one really comes to know the will of God)*. There are some people who surmise that the first thought or voice that comes *after* prayer must belong to the Lord. They do not know how easily Satan can play his trick on them at that moment and lead them astray. There are other people who fancy that the thought or voice which comes *during* prayer must come from God. How about those wandering and wanton thoughts that sometimes flood our

minds during prayer? Can we acknowledge them as coming from God? Of course not! Hence we cannot assume that all which we hear and think during or right after prayer is coming from the Lord.

Some people conclude that a concrete, tangible answer they receive in prayer must surely be the will of God. For instance, I may ask the Lord to open a way for me to do a certain thing. And lo, the way is opened and everything is ready for me to take action. Under such circumstances as these, most of us would likely think that it must certainly be God's will for us to do it. Now sometimes this may indeed be true; nevertheless, this is still not a perfect indication of divine guidance.

Let us take an instance from God's word as an illustration of what has just been said. The children of Israel had lusted exceedingly in the wilderness for meat. The Scriptures tell us this: "he [God] gave them their request, but sent leanness into their soul" (Ps. 106.15). Did not God hear their prayer in this instance? Had He not then performed a great miracle for them that they might have meat to eat? Yet He also sent leanness into their soul, because they were outside of His will to have lusted as they did in their repeated request for meat. How easily they might have mistakenly interpreted the answer to their prayer as proof of their having asked aright in the will of God—that it was indeed His wish to give them meat—yet failing to realize that their leanness of soul was caused by it.

The same could happen to us. Because we pray in the name of the Lord Jesus, we are heard by the Father. But let us here and now be warned lest we consider answered prayer as evidence of our being in the will of God. Sometimes it is better to ask the Lord not to hear our prayer that we may stand firm in His will.

To recapitulate on this point, let us not indiscriminately think that because we have prayed, that because we have received some idea during prayer, or even that because we have had our prayer concretely answered, we can therefore conclude that we must be in God's will. Rather should we seek to know God's will clearly before we make a move. Again let it be reiterated that we are not saying here that answered prayer is totally undependable; not so; yet what we are saying is that we cannot solely depend on it. Other factors need to be taken into account along with answered prayer.

(10) Do not be so stiff-necked or foolish as to wait for the Lord's chastening before knowing His will. Many children of God are frequently out of communion with Him. When their "wild nature" is stirred, they walk according to their own mind. Seeing their wantonness, God is forced to use trial, affliction, even disaster to turn them back. Unless they witness the strong hand of God upon their life, they will not stop proceeding on their own independent way. If, for example, they decide to go somewhere, they will commence their journey without having first ascertained the will of God. They are those who have to wait till they are faced with a mountain without trail or a river without a bridge before they realize that God has not wanted them to go. In doing things they invariably fail to ask the Lord for His will on matters. They will not desist till they

meet the heavy hand of God, either in being laid aside sick, in experiencing a surprising lack of funds, or encountering unexpected disaster. Such believers are to be most pitied.

We can use Balaam and Jonah once again as examples here. Not till he met the angel with the sword drawn did Balaam realize that his trip was not in God's will (see Num. 22.31–34). He thought he could gain fame and wealth by taking this trip to Balak. So, too, in the case of Jonah: not till he was buried in the belly of the great fish did he repent (see Jonah 2). If we possess an instructed heart to seek the Lord's will in all things, we will be saved from many rough and unnecessary encounters in life. How many are the trials, afflictions and sorrows that can thus be avoided! Due to our stubbornness or foolishness, however, these things come our way. Yet let us not think that such behavior and consequences belong only to a certain special group of believers. On the contrary, let us acknowledge that in our own experiences many times we, too, will not desist till God raises His hand against us.

"I will instruct thee and teach thee in the way which thou shalt go: I will counsel thee with mine eye upon thee. Be ye not as the horse, or as the mule, which have no understanding; whose trappings must be bit and bridle to hold them in, else they will not come near unto thee" (Ps. 32.8–9). These two Scripture verses plainly tell us that God's *original* thought is not to instruct us with a strong or heavy hand. He does not want us to be ignorant like the horse or the mule which must be held in with bit and bridle; otherwise, like them, we will not know how to obey. His desire is to have us commune with Him, and through such sweet communion come to know His will and then do it. He promises to guide us with His eye, which means that we ought always to look at Him so as to preclude His having to open His mouth but can counsel us with His eye alone. How wonderful this must be! However, for the Lord to be able to counsel us solely with His eye, we must maintain such communion with Him that as soon as He commands we know instantly and follow immediately. We ought to so wait on Him, look at Him and obey Him that He finds no need to use bit and bridle for getting us to know His will.

Concluding Words

The ten points discussed above are the key elements upon which all who desire to walk in the will of the Lord must take special care to ponder. Please notice that in seeking to walk in the Lord's will we need to consider a variety of factors and not depend on but one particular way or method of guidance; otherwise, we shall fail in our attempt. In the event we make any decision before we are very clear of the Lord's will, we should purpose in our heart to stop proceeding or to change our mind as soon as we discover it is not the will of God. But if we already know of the Lord's will, we must not doubt or hesitate but rather press on and obey to the end, in spite of many oppositions or persecutions seemingly waiting to push us down. In so doing, we will discover that the afflictions and oppositions we anticipate are but the volleys lobbed at us by Satan ahead of time. In that case we can view them as empty threatenings; for as we move on in fulfilling the Lord's will they shall all disappear. Then we shall realize how meaningless have been our fears and doubts.

Hence after clearly knowing the Lord's will, we must launch straight ahead and be anxious for nothing. Though on the way there may be many threats, we nonetheless recognize that these are but the roarings of Satan. They cannot hurt anyone. Therefore, brethren, "Arise, and let us go on!"

11 | How to Know the Will of God*

In his lifetime a Christian has but one occupation, which is to do the will of God so as to obtain eternal joy. If he fails to do so, his future will undoubtedly be gloomy and defective. To many believers, however, their problem lies not in their lack of desire to do God's will, but often in "How do I know the will of God?". The following message, which is based on the Scriptures and spiritual experiences, intends to solve this problem. It is not an impossible task to know God's will. If deep in our heart we really are will-

---

*This article was written in Chinese by the author and published in that language in two parts, appearing in the February and June 1925 issues of the *Spiritual Light* magazine. It is here translated and published in English for the first time. The reader may wish to compare this lengthier discussion of the subject with a briefer but quite similar one the author delivered in message form as one of the now well-known Basic Lesson Series (for new believers) that he gave over two decades later at the Second Workers Training Session held at Mount Kuling in 1949. It can be found in translated form in Volume 4 of the Series, *Not I But Christ* by Watchman Nee (New York: Christian Fellowship Publishers, 1974), pp. 125–43, and entitled "The Will of God."—*Translator*

*ing to obey His will, we shall unquestionably have it
clearly revealed to us.—Ruth Lee**

Introduction

We invariably notice that an architect will have a
prepared blueprint for the construction of an edifice.
He draws a detailed plan for the new structure he is
going to build. Everything about the edifice—its size,
large or small, its height, tall or low—is minutely
planned. During the time of construction, all is done
according to his plan. In the building of all modern
edifices, every one of them will have had the pre-laid
plans of the architect drawn up.

When the children of Israel built the tabernacle in
the wilderness, they too had a preconceived plan. They
did not set about building a tabernacle for Jehovah on
a mere whim. Moses received instruction from God,
who not only showed him on Mount Sinai the pattern
of the tabernacle but also explained to him each item
in detail. He was ordered to build on earth a tabernacle
that was according to what had been revealed to him
from heaven. And hence, in the building of this tent
structure, there was first the plan and then the construction. Every minute detail of the tabernacle had been
decided upon by God in advance. Even the material for
such a tiny thing as a pin was disclosed to Moses by
God. Furthermore, Moses had no authority to alter at
will the smallest item in the tabernacle. The entire struc-

---

*Editor, at the time, of *Spiritual Light* magazine, and later a close
associate of Watchman Nee.—*Translator*

ture with all its parts was entirely planned by God for His chosen people to build accordingly.

A man's life and his daily work are all planned by God. He has His definite plan for the lifework and daily activities of every believer. He has His perfect will towards all His blood-bought ones. He has designed beforehand the movements of His regenerated children. Since God the Father has His scheme for them, He expects Christians to follow carefully what He has laid out.

Ignorant construction laborers who follow their own thoughts and not the well-laid plan of the architect are doomed to fail in their building work. In like manner, how could the work of the children of Israel ever be acceptable to God the Master Architect if they did not erect the tabernacle in accordance with the direction He had given them? Likewise, Christians who do not follow the pre-determined plan of God for their lives are destined to fall. Violation of God's will is the root of all failure of believers.

A very important question arises here. "How can we know the will of God?" Many believers consider themselves not as those who do not love to do God's will but as those who do love to do His will. Yet they do not do His will because they do not know what His will is. We are therefore not concerned here with those who are careless about God's will but concerned with those who single-heartedly desire to do God's will. And many of them have a major problem in "How to know the will of God." I know very well that many brothers and sisters in the Lord have this difficulty. They have already consecrated themselves to God; they sincerely expect the pleasure and approval of God. They love to do His will. Yet they have no idea what constitutes His will concerning their lives and works. They do not know what is the will of God towards certain matters; they are groping in darkness; consequently, they cannot but err. Many tears are shed and many hearts are broken because of this deficiency in knowledge. How painful is such an experience! Nonetheless, there is one thing we ought to know:

God Is Responsible for Letting Us Know His Will

This is something easily understood. For if God wants us to do His will, He should tell us what that will is. How can He possibly expect us to live and work in agreement with His will if He fails to inform us what that will is? In the event of our failure because He has not revealed His mind to us, He himself must bear the responsibility. To reveal to us His will is what God ought to do. For example, a father wants his son to do a certain thing on a certain day, but he fails to share his thought with his son. When that day arrives, his son continues to perform his usual duties without carrying out the special thing that has been upon his father's heart. Which of these two do you judge should be responsible? The son? No! It is the father. Since the father has not informed the son of his will, how can the latter be responsible for not doing that will? If the father wants his son to do something for him, he should tell the son of his will.

Now our heavenly Father is most kind to us. Whenever He wants us to do His will, He always tells it to us beforehand. In the parable of the two sons which our Lord Jesus himself has narrated, the father wanted his sons to go work in the vineyard. So he told them his desire. The son who later did what was commanded was obedient, while the son who did not carry out the father's order was deemed rebellious (see Matt. 21.28–31). We thank God our Father, for He always discloses His secret plan to us.

Not Knowing God's Will—Our Fault

We acknowledge that God always tells us what He requires of us that we may know His will. Yet in our experiences, is it not true that many times we wish to know God's will but we simply are unable to know? Why is this so? Since God is willing to inform us of His will, why is it that many times we find ourselves unable to discern it? Since on God's side there is the need of letting us know His will, and yet we fail to perceive it, the problem must be on the side of us believers. There must be some obstacle to the possibility of God revealing His will to us. Abraham was always obedient to the Lord. So when God thought of destroying Sodom and Gomorrah, the Scriptures tell us this: "And Jehovah said, Shall I hide from Abraham that which I do … ?" (Gen. 18.17) In order for God to reveal His will, nothing must stand between us and Him. Otherwise, even though He wants to show us His will, we are not able to receive, because we do not have an open heart. God may reveal, but we can neither see nor hear nor understand. To be in tune with God is an essential requirement for knowing His will.

The Conditions for Knowing God's Will

In order to know the Lord's will, the matter of first importance is to cast aside our own opinion. This is because our preconceived idea frequently hinders God from being able to disclose His will to us. Such prejudice shuts the will of God out of our heart. I must confess that in my own personal experiences, whenever I failed to know the will of God, invariably it was because I already had had my own idea (sometimes my own thought was hidden in the depth of my heart). Unless I got rid of my self idea, I could encounter many difficulties in seeking to know the Lord's will. But soon after I laid it aside, God would be able to show me His will.

This matter of getting rid of our self idea as a prerequisite for knowing God's will is so essential that I can never overemphasize it. This point is so important that great attention must be given to it. Let me therefore discuss the matter further.

How deceitful is our heart. Sometimes we may appear to be seeking the will of God, yet within our hearts we are filled with self idea and personal opinion, for our one dominating desire is to please ourselves. Sometimes as we kneel to pray, our mouth may say, "O Lord, may You reveal Your will to me, for I am willing to do Your will." But in actuality, our heart neither approves nor wills to do His will. Sometimes we may pray, "O Father, may Your will be done. I only seek after Your will." Our heart seems to be agreeing with our mouth that we earnestly desire to do God's will. Nonetheless, in the depth of our hearts there exists another desire to seek our own will. In such a state as this, we will probably never get to know God's will. Any false seeking will never make any real gain. For the promise of "seek and ye shall find" (Matt. 7.7) is not given to a dishonest heart. Except we really seek after God's will, we shall not be given revelation of that will. Even if we should comfort ourselves by saying, "I already know God's will," this most likely is the product of our own thought—which is a counterfeit of His will.

If there is already secret desire in us, it is in vain to seek the Lord's will. Having our own idea, none of our prayers will avail anything. Even if we pray daily to know God's will, these prayers will prove to be totally futile. For this reason, each time we wish to seek the will of the Lord, we should examine ourselves before Him to see if there is any self idea in the depth of our heart, if there is any inclination, any secret self-centered longing. Seek His will with a pure and undefiled heart; else all is useless.

Let us suppose that there are two ways (or even more) before you: one is the way on which you would like to travel; the other is the way or path on which you would not like to travel. Doubtless you will ask yourself, "If the Lord commands me to go the way I do not like, will I be willing to obey?" In case you are not willing to obey, what then is the benefit of knowing the will of the Lord?

Whenever we are faced with diverging roads, the best is for us to have no inclination at all, which means we maintain a balanced heart, looking at the roads ahead with the same attitude, neither loving one road or fearful of the other. With such an attitude as this in us, it shall be most easy for the Lord to reveal His will to us. On the other hand, having any set inclination or harboring an unwillingness to obey becomes the greatest obstruction to knowing the will of the Lord. To have no inclination does not mean putting ourselves in a passive mood. It is related to the road ahead of us. We ought to exercise our will in deciding to do God's will. Hence to say that there is no inclination in our heart does not imply that we do not even have the desire of knowing. It only suggests that before we know the will of God we have no bending towards either road. But we are determined that once we know His will we will do it. So far as our own wish is concerned, we have no "like" or "dislike" at all towards the roads before us. Yet even before we know God's will, we have made a choice between His will and our will; which is, that we have decided for God's will as against our own. We choose His will and reject our own. Therefore, we are not without will and without choice. We do have them, but they are on the side of God's will. We want what the Lord wants.

We may learn this very lesson from the life of our Lord Jesus Christ. The human will of our Lord and the will of the heavenly Father are not one but two wills. When we read: "Nevertheless not my will, but thine, be done" (Luke 22.42b), we can conclude with certainty that the will of the Lord Jesus and that of God the Father are separate realities. There is this word of Scripture also: "I seek not mine own will, but the will of him that sent me" (John 5.30b). This clearly shows that these two wills are indeed distinguishable.

However, even though the will of the Lord Jesus and

the will of the Father came from two separate sources, nonetheless we notice that there was no controversy between them. For in spite of the fact that our gracious Lord had His own will, He nevertheless laid aside His own to do His Father's will. He placed His own will on the side of God. He willed to obey the Father. He did not passively do God's will; rather, He actively laid down His will that He might do the Father's will. He denied His own will and desired the Father's. And thus His will was none other than doing the Father's will. Formerly, His will differed from the Father's. But now He willed to do the Father's will which heretofore was different from His. For this reason the whole life of our Lord is well-pleasing to God the Father.

To sum up, then, this first step in our seeking the Lord's will, we must not harbor in our heart any like or dislike towards the roads ahead of us before we know which of these is the will of God. Yet at the same time we must maintain an attitude of desiring to do God's will. In the event of our willingness to submit our will to the will of the Lord, our seeking to know His will is already half done. The reason why we fail to know the Lord's will is largely due to failure on this very point. To the one who wills to do the Lord's will, he shall of course be shown what that will is. But to him who does not will that will, his seeking after the Lord's will is false; and the will of the Lord is not to be given to such a person. Therefore, if there is already a set inclination in your heart, do not pretend to say that you want to know the will of the Lord. You should first deal with your own heart desire and inclination by the power of God. Then you will receive the revelation of His will.

Otherwise, knowing and using all the methods of seeking after God's will shall result in nothing.

Having submitted our will to the Lord, we have gotten rid of this fundamental obstacle so that God cannot help but reveal His will to us.

How God Causes Us to Know His Will

There are altogether three methods. We must not look solely to one such method. For if we do so, we can easily fall into Satan's snares. We must look at and follow all three together, and thus shall we be saved from lopsidedness. Having perfect light, we may walk in God's will perfectly. These three methods are: the inspiration of the Holy Spirit, the teaching of the Scriptures, and the provision of environment. On one occasion when on shipboard, Dr. F. B. Meyer asked the ship's captain, as the ship approached the waters to London, "In this vast ocean, how do you know this entry into port is the correct one?" The captain replied, "As I navigate the ship to the position where those three lighthouses ahead form one straight line, then I know I have safely arrived at London harbor." Just so, Dr. Meyer wrote, "When we see the Holy Spirit, the Holy Scriptures, and environment—these three—agree in one, then I know I am in the will of God." Indeed, the agreement of these three proves that we stand in the will of God.

(1) THE INSPIRATION OF THE HOLY SPIRIT

There is no one in the world who does things entirely according to his own will, since if he is not doing *God's* will he shall invariably be doing the *devil's.* "In the sons of disobedience," writes Paul, "the prince of the powers of the air" is working (Eph. 2.2). In those who obey the Lord, "it is God who worketh in [them] both to will and to work" (Phil. 2.13). It can therefore be said that in a person's heart, either the evil spirit is at work or else God is. None of us on earth can be exempt from either of these two workings. Whoever the person is, each of his actions is either the result of the working of the Holy Spirit in him or that of the evil spirit. Even a believer is not able to escape completely from this situation.

Whenever a person does anything, he is moved to do it. Sometimes he may be deeply moved; at other times he may be only slightly moved. And as a consequence of this kind of inspiration or impulse in his heart, he sets to work.

What is most lamentable is that believers generally are ignorant of the life in the Holy Spirit as well as of the Holy Spirit in their lives. As their soul is becoming stirred they may quite easily reckon this to be the movement of the Holy Spirit. They are unable to distinguish the inspiration of the Holy Spirit from the incitement of the soul. Is it not in fact quite difficult to discern what is the incitement of the soul and what is the inspiration of the Holy Spirit? For young Christians, of course, this is naturally hard; but the matured saints can easily separate them as a child is able to differentiate between wheat and tares.

Now besides the confusion caused by the mixing of soulical incitement and the Spirit's inspiration, there can also be the deception in believers caused by the devil who frequently fashions himself as an angel of light and even feigns the voice of the Holy Spirit. Let us not imagine that all which Satan has plotted for us is necessarily all bad, dirty and mean. Let us realize that his chief motive is to lead us from the will of God. Indeed, he sometimes (perhaps even quite often) leads the believers to do good things so as to make them think that good things are God's will. Who can understand this truth: that although God's will is always good, good things may not always be God's will? Satan is not afraid of Christians doing good things; he is only fearful of their doing the will of God. As long as he is able to entice believers away from doing God's will, he is fully satisfied. For this reason, whenever a believer wishes to know the will of God, let him not conclude under some kind of incitement that because a certain thing is good, it is therefore bound to be God's will. For not all good things are God's will; and even if they are, who knows whether they are God's foreordained will for *you* or for *me?*

Hence regarding the inspiration of the Holy Spirit in relation to seeking to know the will of God, three things need to be distinguished: (a) the inspiration of the Holy Spirit, (b) the incitement of the soul, and (c) the instigation of Satan. The first is a kind of movement of the Spirit of God in our spirit which causes us to know His will. Such movement or inspiration is *quiet* and *sustained,* not *sudden* and *exciting.* It belongs to God. The apostle Paul once asserted, "I go bound in the *spirit* unto Jerusalem" (Acts 20.22a). Let us also read these words about Paul: "Now while Paul waited for them at Athens, his *spirit* was provoked within him as he beheld the city full of idols. So he reasoned in the synagogue with the Jews and the devout persons, and in the marketplace every day with them that met him" (Acts. 17.16-17). The Holy Spirit inspired Paul, causing his spirit to feel as though bound without any freedom. The same Spirit of God also provoked Paul's spirit to preach as though some sort of power worked in him and caused him to obey.

How very sad that believers do not even know what the "spirit" is. They are unaware that man is a tripartite being of spirit, soul and body (see 1 Thess. 5.23). What they know is that a man has a soul and a body. Many believers may recognize in letter "spirit" and "soul," and they may even acknowledge that besides the Holy Spirit there is the human spirit. Yet in their lives they do not feel as though they have a spirit. They are totally ignorant of the activities within them —whether these are the operations of the Spirit or the rousings of the soul. Some carelessly interpret soul to be spirit! Now due to such lack of accurate knowledge, they find it most difficult to know the will of God.

Some believers commit the error of regarding "mind" as spirit. But "mind" belongs to the soul; it does not belong to the human spirit. The thoughts of the mind are untrustworthy and should not be accepted as the inspiration of the Holy Spirit.

We have already described a little the phenomena of the inspiration of the Holy Spirit. For the sake of weak or immature children of God, we may add a few more words here. The inspiration of the Holy Spirit usually gives us faith; that is to say, that when God wants you to do a certain thing, He will grant you a firm faith, you firmly believing that what you are about to do is of God's will. Such firm belief comes to you in *quietness.* And when this firm belief is given, a quiet peace enters your heart as a fresh anointing. This firm belief, however, needs to be supported by faith. Then it will never rebel: it will neither be affected by changing circumstances nor troubled with doubting God's will. For the beginners in the Christian life it is essential always to remember that the inspiration of the Holy Spirit is *powerful* yet *quiet, gradual* and never *compulsive.* God always waits for the consent of your free will to obey and follow His and lets *you* do it. He never oppresses you with a kind of force as though to *overwhelm* you. Another thing to keep in mind is this: that the inspiration of the Holy Spirit always comes from *within,* since God works from the center to the circumference. He usually operates first in the human spirit that in turn enlightens the mind of the soul to cause it to understand. Only after the approval of the believer himself shall God's will be finally wrought out in the body in the act of obedience.

The incitement of the soul, on the other hand, is a sort of emotional activity. Sometimes, due to some special reason, you feel elated and pleased. At such a time you think of many things to do. Moreover, your emotional power seems to be so high that you also cannot leave a thing undone. In order to distinguish what is the soul's incitement and what is the Spirit's inspiration, we would do well to remember a few rules. Incitement is usually governed by environment. When we are alone by ourselves, we experience a certain sensation.

Whatever incitement induces us to do always comes *suddenly*. There seems to be a fire within us that overwhelms us. Our heart is not quiet but may be burning and confused. If we are able to stop proceeding and to let that excited emotion ebb away, we shall soon discover that the thing we were incited to do that day was not the will of God. Here is one thing we may discern: that *the feeling* we have when incited is all in our *emotion*. There is not that firm belief within our heart. God, on the other hand, is patient. He through the Spirit is never in haste in what He does. He spoke once through the prophet Isaiah, saying: "He that believeth shall not be in haste" (Is. 28.16). Hence, when by the Holy Spirit He inspires us, God takes time. Sudden feeling is nine times out of ten not an indication of His will.

The instigation of Satan and the inspiration of the Holy Spirit are so opposite in practice that they are virtually antagonistic to each other. Nevertheless, because of their similar appearance many believers find it difficult to discern the one from the other. For Satan does not always cause us to commit sin. What he often aims at is to lead us out of and away from God's will. Sometimes he hinders us so that we lag behind God's will; at other times he pushes us to go overboard ahead of God's will. He fashions himself as an angel of light feigning the voice of the Spirit of God. He will whisper in our ears that which will cause us to be confused about the still, small voice of the Holy Spirit.

Now children of God need to be exercised to differentiate Satan's *suggestion* from the Holy Spirit's *revelation*. The Enemy's instigation always comes *suddenly*. He uses a "blitzlike" strategy against Christians.

The inspiration of the Holy Spirit, however, is first revelation followed by an enlightening of the mind. Satan's first work is to *inject* a seed thought into the believer's mind. Such thought arrives suddenly and carries with it many reasons. He first creates numerous reasonings and many methods in the believer's mind before he causes him to do a certain thing. Because there are many reasons, believers frequently mistake these to be the inspiration of the Holy Spirit. Yet whereas the latter always works *from within,* such seed thought usually enters *from without.* Therefore, the children of God must not accept *sudden* thought as constituting the will of God. We should be careful and steady. Before doing anything, we must resolve all doubts. We need to be cautious towards all sudden instigations from outside, because nine-tenths of them are not the inspiration of the Holy Spirit.

(2) The Teaching of the Scriptures

Having understood the inspiration of the Holy Spirit, God's children should also know the teaching of the Scriptures on different matters. This is important for safety's sake. The teaching of the Scriptures in view here does not have reference to the teaching of a certain verse of a certain chapter—that is to say, the taking of a text out of context. This latter practice many believers engage in in time of need. They will read a verse or two in the Bible, and then take these as God's foreordained will for them. Or on other occasions, and after earnest prayer, they will open the Bible at random and read a few verses. If the word happens to fit in with their circumstances, they consider it to be God's will. Their action or inaction, coming or going, will be decided by these few verses. On the other hand, if the word found there at random has no relevance to their situation but is at least not contradictory to it, they will not interpret is as being no guidance from God. On the contrary, they will try to twist these random verses to make it adaptable to their circumstances, condition or situation so as to enable them to decide their future action. Such a method of approach to the teaching of the Bible is highly dangerous. How impossible it is to expect guidance from the Scriptures about which one has no knowledge!

What, then, do we mean by knowing the teaching of the Scriptures in the believer's life? Let us see that it points to the *unified* testimony of the *whole* Bible. In other words, we must see how the entire Bible teaches on any given subject or situation. How does it speak on the thing a person intends to do? We need to understand what the Old Testament says and what the New Testament says. We need also to know how things were resolved in the time of the Patriarchs, under the law, and now under grace. For what we now obey is not the judgment of the *Old* Covenant, but that of the *New:* not the Patriarchs, nor the decision of the Law, but the command of *grace.*

Will this make it really difficult? Who can understand except those exalted Bible scholars? Hence this is one of the reasons why we all of us must search the Scriptures. What the Bible records is God's will for the entire world, for people living under ancient and modern dispensations. If believers want to know the will of God, they must study (not just read) the Bible. And the words of the Bible are *easily* understood, for according to the Lord Jesus himself they are revealed to babes (see Matt. 11.25). The Scriptures are God's complete revelation. It has clear exposition on His plan, precept, purpose and all kinds of problems. God gives the Bible to His own people in anticipation of their being able to understand all His will. Consequently, there is no excuse for a believer who does not study the Bible to then say that he does not know God's will.

Perhaps at times when a problem is too big or too complicated for you to really know what the Bible teaches, you can seek help from a more spiritually exercised Christian. The Lord is able to use such a person to instruct you. Yet you should not overly rely on another person's word. You yourself ought to *discern* what he has said to you (see 1 Cor. 14.29), and then decide if the answer is in accordance with the word of the Scriptures. If we ourselves do not search the Scriptures, and if we are unwilling to ask another believer who is more spiritual, but instead we randomly turn to one or two Scripture verses and accept them as an indication of God's will and thereafter carry it out, our failure will predictably be sure.

The importance of obeying the word of the Scriptures is clearly demonstrated in the temptations the first and the Last Adam encountered, respectively, in the Garden of Eden and in the wilderness. One Adam suffered defeat while the Other could claim victory. The deciding factor of victory or defeat lay in none other fact than that the first Adam did not obey God's word whereas the Last Adam did obey it. The defeat suffered in the Garden of Eden because of disobeying God's word has become the root cause of all human rebellion. In the wilderness, however, the Last Adam, even our Lord Jesus Christ, overcame the Enemy and his temptations three successive times by His obedience to the word of the Scriptures. At that time the devil's temptations appeared to be quite innocent, even very sympathetic in character; but the Lord kept the word of the Scriptures with fear and trembling. And hence He won the perfect victory. As a result, it is now possible for the rule of *our* daily life to be essentially the Holy Scriptures. If we seek the teaching of the Bible in all things, we will not walk outside the will of God.

Consequently, after we are moved by the Holy Spirit, we need to ask if this inward motion is one with the Scriptures. This is because we are not sure if what we have been inspired to do is really of the Holy Spirit. By such asking and searching, the truth of the matter will be demonstrated one way or the other. For the Holy Scriptures are inspired by the Holy Spirit and they reveal the will of God. It is absolutely impossible for the Holy Spirit to say one thing in the Holy Scriptures and say another thing in us. The inspiration of the Holy Spirit and the teaching of the Holy Scriptures are *forever* the same and *never* contradictory to each other. As a matter of fact, the Holy Spirit and the Holy Scriptures work together in revealing to us the right path. They unite in telling us the will of God. They never differ in their directions. In the event anyone declares he has been moved by the Holy Spirit to do a certain thing and yet that thing is opposed by the Scriptures, his professed inspiration is undoubtedly false. May we remember this well, that when inspiration and Scripture disagree, let us be quiet and not act. We had always better check to see if the inspiration comes from the Holy Spirit, and if so, to see further, if it is one with the Scriptures.

Sometimes, however, the Scriptures may not seem to have any bearing on doing or not doing, going or not going. For example, if you want to go and preach in a certain place, such *going* is Scriptural because there is already much plain teaching in the Bible which demonstrates God's approval of our evangelizing the gospel. But *not* going is not necessarily wrong, either, since the Scriptures also record how on a few occasions the Lord forbade His apostles at certain *times* to go to places to preach (see Acts 16.6–7). Under such circumstances, the important thing to do is to discern carefully the Holy Spirit's inspiration and its attraction. If the Spirit gives a definite leading, you may go.

(3) THE PROVISION OF ENVIRONMENT

Environment frequently serves as a good instrument in expressing God's will. This does not have reference to the approval or opposition of men. It denotes God's provision in our personal environment. Being in God's will does not preclude us from being misunderstood and opposed by many people. Not because there is man's opposition, therefore such circumstance indicates that we should not go to a certain place or do a certain thing. Not so. We learn from the Bible how the apostles of the Early Church were attacked by the people and how they were jailed many times. Their environment was truly adverse to them. Yet did they not walk in the will of God? They themselves said to the Jewish High Council at Jerusalem: "Whether it is right in the sight of God to hearken unto you rather than unto God, judge ye: for we cannot but speak the things which we saw and heard" (Acts 4.19–20). Again they said, "We must obey God rather than men" (Acts 5.29). They listened to God, and they were in His will. Consequently, for us to say that environment can be an instrument to express God's will cannot have reference to the environment which men may have provided us. In the works of God, people's antagonism is often at the instigation of Satan. Hence this is not to be considered. Apart from the people, God must make provisions for us personally for the work He calls us to do. He will provide all our needs — physical strength, adequate finance, and sometimes natural assistance to help us on.

The hand of God is frequently shown in environment. He often is behind our daily happenings. A matured Christian can see the moving of the Lord's hand in his environments. For He is the God of all things. He is the source of all things as well as the end of all things. Blessed is the believer who has learned to seek God's will in his environment. A consecrated believer resists on the one hand what comes from Satan and accepts on the other whatever circumstances the Lord has arranged for him. We know that without God's permission, nothing can fall upon us. This we gather from the Book of Job. Although Satan is the prime mover of all disasters, he is nonetheless controlled by God from behind. For all his activities are under Heaven's restraint. In the Bible we can find many incidents wherein God's hand was at the control. These include the smallest things as well as the biggest ones. For He is not only the Lord of big things, He is also the Lord of small things. If the very hairs of the believers are numbered, is there anything not in the hand of God? Blessed are those who know Romans 8.28 which says, "We know that to them that love God all things work together for good, even to them that are called according to purpose."

Hence after he has known the inspiration of the Holy Spirit and the teaching of the Scriptures a believer should also see how God will provide in his environment. If He wants you to do a certain thing, He without fail will give you the opportunity, time, and strength (both physical and spiritual) to do it. He will also provide you with fellow-workers if you need them. He will certainly provide all that you need; for is not one of His names "Jehovah-jireh" — "Jehovah will provide!" (see Gen. 22.14 mgn). If you are truly in the will of God, you will see many so-called *coincidences*. You will be surprised at the many "accidental" sequences of events that appear to have a causal relationship along your way. These are not "coincidences" or "casual happenings" but are the *orderings* of God. He causes all things to come together to meet our needs. Accordingly, all who walk in the will of God have no need to strive against the things which come from outside, for the Lord is using them to be the steps to success for His servants and maids. Even if men's oppositions cannot be avoided, He will provide every need.

The above three methods are the ways God uses to express himself. Each time He guides His children, He employs these three methods. The agreement of these three proves to the believers whether or not they are in the will of God. The Holy Spirit, the Holy Scriptures, and environment must not contradict one another. In the event of contradiction, we can judge the matter as not being God's will. Let believers well remember these three methods as they seek to walk before God.

Special Situations

Sometimes the situation may be very peculiar. There may be two conflicting thoughts in our mind as though either doing or not doing is the will of God; in other words, it is hard to decide which is right and which is wrong. Furthermore, the Scriptures may seem to be neutral on the subject, opposing neither of them. Even the environment might appear to be open to both actions. In such a situation, the best way is to maintain an attitude of withstanding Satan. If we truly desire to do God's will, we at this juncture should take a firm stand of approving all that is of the Lord and opposing all that is of Satan. Though we are yet unsure which is of God and which is of the Enemy, we can nonetheless maintain an attitude of wanting what God wants and denying what is not His. At the same time we can pray: "O God, I want what is Yours; I do not want what is not Yours. Please show me what is Yours and what is not." With such sincere desire for God's will as this, we shall soon be shown what is His and what is not His. God will enable us to know for sure. We cannot overemphasize this point, since it is quite important.

Sometimes Satan will so disturb us that we falter between two ways. Yet if we affirm our attitude of approving God's heart and opposing Satan, our confusion will either immediately vanish or soon disappear. However, before we are given to know the will of God, the best prescription is the following:

No Knowledge, No Action

Wait patiently before the Lord, willing to act only after His will is known. For sometimes when God considers that it is profitable for us to know His will a little later, He will delay in revealing it to us. During such time, we should maintain the attitude of *no knowledge, no action.* The psalmist once said: "Neither do I exercise myself in great matters, or in things too wonderful for me" (Ps. 131.1b). Hence, at the time of not knowing the mystery, we would rather not act, lest we find it necessary to repent later on. Many faults and repentance are due to acting in haste. Our danger lies in being too active, in that before we know the Lord's will, we have already taken action. The Lord wants us to wait on Him and move forward at His step. Only after we truly know God's will do we begin to move our hands and feet. How sad that we frequently are pressed by environment to act hastily, thus running away from God's will. It is accurate to state that nine out of ten times things hastily done are not of God's will. When the Lord Jesus was on earth He never did anything in haste. We should imitate Him. Before we are one hundred percent sure of the Lord's will, we should never take any presumptuous actions. We are determined only to begin after knowing God's will.

Sometimes under excitement or stimulation we may promise to do a certain thing, but we realize afterwards that it is not the will of the Lord. What should we do then? Speaking in Psalm 15 about "them that feareth Jehovah," the word of God goes on to assert that whoever among them "sweareth to his own hurt, and changeth not ... shall never be moved" (vv. 4b,5b). These verses refer to those who are already believers. Believers ought to treat people in righteousness: "Yea, yea; nay, nay" (Matt. 5.37); and "not yea and nay" (2 Cor. 1.19b). In the light of God's Scriptures, we cannot go back on our word once given or promised. But when we find ourselves in such a situation just described, we can only confess before the Lord that our promise has been faulty and ask Him to so work as to make that promise ineffective. The Lord will open a way out. Yet if the Lord has some other purpose for our mistake, we must learn to submit. Though it is a cursed thing to act wrongly, nonetheless, we do read that "Jehovah thy God turned the curse into a blessing unto thee" (Deut. 23.5b). Hence wait upon the Lord with great patience.

Thus Be Delivered from Many Troubles

Many things in which we are busily engaged prove to be empty because they are not in God's will. If what we do is outside of His will, the Lord whom we serve will not be pleased. We may be busy from dawn to dusk, yet if our works have no spiritual benefit, we will not receive God's praise and reward. We will be saved from many meaningless "busynesses" if we determine not to act in any or all of them before we know the will of

God in relation to them. This will deliver us from being busy all day long so that we may have more time to be quiet before the Lord and commune with Him.

Small Things

We should seek the Lord's will in all our daily affairs. If we carelessly follow our own will in the *small* things of the day, we will find ourselves distant from the Lord when we try to seek His will in the *big* things. In that case His will shall appear to us as "yea and nay." Though we may spend much time in seeking, we are still frustrated. Because of this, we ought to seek the Lord's will equally in the small matters as in the large ones. If we are accustomed to know the Lord's will daily, we shall find no trouble in knowing His will when special things happen. We should be so exercised in habitually knowing God's will that we may know and follow it whenever any matter comes our way.

Nevertheless, Satan is so cunning that once he realizes a believer is seeking God's will in all things, he will suggest many small things to the believer's mind as the wills of God. And what things he suggests along this line are mostly abnormal in character. For example, he will suggest that you should take a crooked path which is both longer and more difficult instead of taking the straight and main road which you would ordinarily take. There can be many things like that. Within a single day the Enemy may falsify God's will and tell you many, many things. At such time, you should maintain an attitude of resisting Satan as we have said before. We ought to investigate if these are the wills of God.

This is because sometimes, for a special reason, God may order us to go around the regular path in order to protect us. Remember that although the Lord has His will in all things, He never abolishes man's reasoning power. For those whose minds have been renewed, the Spirit of God will, in the small things (except in very special cases), lead us by our rational power; so that in many small things, we need not be deceived by Satan if we are faithful to exercise our normal, rational power of discernment. Sometimes Satan may accuse us for not following his counterfeit will. This we must resist. (Notice that this section of the message has been dealing only with small things).

Seek and Do

In seeking to know the will of God, we must have an honest heart to do what we know. True seeking ends in doing. The reason for seeking to *know* is to *do* God's will. Otherwise, what is the purpose and benefit of knowing? Knowing but not doing His will is sinning against God. It only nourishes our flesh and causes it to live. The flesh always sees the hardship of God's will; therefore, it lays back and is afraid to proceed. Unless we put to death the deeds of the flesh and do the will of God, our spiritual life will suffer a serious blow. The Lord wants us to *do* His will, not just to *know* it. He shows us His will that we may do it. Not doing is hollow knowing! God loves to see us doing His will. True knowledge is demonstrated by our doing.

Here let us reiterate that in our heart there must not be any self-inclination, self-opinion, or secret desire;

otherwise, we will not be given to know God's will. If we are not willing to do His will, He is also unwilling to show us His will. Having a willing heart to do God's will, we shall naturally be shown it. Yet the children of God frequently have one problem, which is, that there is

A Natural Desire in the Heart

On this matter of doing God's will, it seems as though personal inclination, secret desire and self-will naturally exist. We feel it is too costly, too much against our own will to follow His will. It makes our flesh suffer and our feeling uncomfortable. This does not necessarily indicate that we have no desire to know God's will. On the contrary, we may love to know, but in our heart there is also that self-desire. How can we be delivered from such a mixed condition? On the one hand, we need to acknowledge God's rights over us more and more. We should meditate on the love of Christ — how He died for us, how much He suffered, how He saved us and showed mercy towards us. In view of His rights, we ought to obey Him. In view of His love, we are constrained to follow Him. We consider Him till our hearts are melted and our tears flow. If we do this, then without fail the love of Christ will move us.

On the other hand, we could ask ourselves: "Originally I did not like to do God's will, for I had my own inclination. Am I now willing to let Him make me willing and take away my own inclination?" In other words, we may not be directly willing to do God's will, yet are we willing to be *in*directly made willing by Him?

Or to put it in still another way, though we ourselves do not have the willingness to do God's will, will we let Him change our unwillingness into willingness? If we do not have the first willingness, do we have the second willingness? In the event we have neither the willingness to do God's will nor the willingness to let Him make us willing, it is certain that we will not know God's will. (What would be the use even if we did know?!) Ultimately we must fall through our self-will. Nevertheless, even if we have not the direct willingness but have the indirect willingness, God will surely work in our spirit as well as in our environment to make us willing.

How amazing it is that the Lord will work the miracle of turning human hearts to make us willing. Sometimes such a step takes time, since God never forces anyone. If we feel we cannot obey Him, nor will we allow Him to make us obey, He will not work at all. What Philippians 2.13 declares is indeed a great truth: "it is God who worketh in you both to will and to work, for his good pleasure." This does not mean that God wills instead of us. It simply means He works in us till we will His will.

For this reason, even if we are not willing to do the Lord's will, we should at least have a willingness to allow Him to transform our unwilling heart. Thus shall He work in our heart and make us willing. But if we do not even have this tiny little willingness in us, then it is beyond any doubt that what we do is outside God's will and unacceptable to Him. How blessed and happy are those who are attracted by the love of God and who await the future glory. In their hearts they are ever ready for God's order and have not the slightest desire of not doing His will.

The Important Question

George Mueller was deeply experienced in prayer and communion with the Lord. He once said that every time he did something, he first asked himself a few questions, among which the most important were: Is this the will of God? Is this God's will for me? Is this His time? Is this His way? He would wait till he clearly knew the answers to all these questions before he decided his action. Here we need to learn from him. Let us be careful, like George Mueller, and we will make no mistake.

Final Word

If we truly offer ourselves entirely to the Lord, we will come to see how He governs our lives. Many things which we reckon as beautiful and appropriate we dare not and will not do because they are not of God's will. Many works which we might consider profitable and lovely, we also will not and dare not do because in *them* we are not given His will. Whatever is not the will of God, even a thought or an idea, we will gladly lay aside. We are determined to do the Lord's will, to please Him and not ourselves. In spite of what we deem precious and desirable, we are willing to lay it down for the Lord's sake. What bondage! Blessed bondage!! What restraint! Blessed restraint!! What inhibition! Blessed inhibition!! Daily we see our own thoughts and opinions dashed to pieces. Daily we meet "frustrations." How beautiful is the restraining hand of the Lord. Our hearts magnify the Lord. He must increase; we must decrease. Our hearts rejoice in seeing ourselves being stripped and the Lord's will being done. May He enable us always to know His will and to do it. "O Lord! When our self is imprisoned and grieved, we are truly joyful, for then Your heart is pleased."

"That ye may stand perfect and fully assured in all the will of God" (Col. 4.12b).

PART TWO

ADMONITION AND DISCIPLINE*

*The twenty-seven short articles of varying length that comprise this Part were written by the author in Chinese and first appeared in published form in the various issues of either *The Christian* magazine for 1925 and 1926 or those of *Spiritual Light* magazine for 1925. Now collected together in trnslated form, they here appear in English for the first time. — *Translator*

Admonition and Discipline

1. *Humility* We know that the heavier the load is, the lower the ship sinks; the weightier the fruits, the more bent the branch; and the bigger the tree, the deeper the root. This also is true with the man who has received much grace. He who receives less grace tends to boast of the little he gets. A humble man is one who is full of God's grace. For God alone can cause one to be humble. Humility is not *thinking* less of oneself, but is thinking of oneself not at all. Humility is not *looking* less at oneself, but is looking at oneself not at all. A truly humble person is one who has truly died to himself. If self is not dead, he will inwardly glorify himself even though he may not show it outwardly. Indeed, the heart of a man is deceitful above all things (see Jer. 17.9).

However, let us see that humility is one thing but timidity is another. These two should not be confused. Man's own humbleness which comes either from natural temperament or from human effort will always lead to timidity. And the final product will be a flight from responsibility. But true humility in the Lord will not hide under the name of modesty and shun any responsibility. For in the things of God, the truly humble man boldly marches forward on the one hand, and on the other he confesses his own weakness and inability so as to depend on God constantly. "In all thy ways acknowledge him" (Prov. 3.6a). Fearful of standing forth is not humility, rather it is a spiritual defect. How very difficult it is to be humble before the Lord and at the same time bear heavy responsibility. Nevertheless, Philippians 4.13 is truly a trustworthy word here: "I can do all things in him that strengtheneth me." Let us therefore look to the Lord.

2. *Obedience* How sweet it is to obey the Lord! How joyful the heart is in losing many things for the sake of obeying the Lord! People who have not traveled the way of obedience and who have never lost anything for the Lord can hardly feel and understand such sweetness and joy. Yet the obedient ones daily consider loss as gain and shame as glory. There is a reward for obeying the Lord, and that reward is having more power to deny self and to obey the Lord again the next time. Disobeying the Lord also has its punishment, which is, a yielding more to self and a rebelling more against the Lord.

Even in this life, the Lord becomes more manifested through our obedience, and joy increases through sufferings due to obedience. How much more would believers honor the Lord if they knew this. Alas, our obedience is so limited in measure! How rare is absolute obedience and yet how sweet it is. In order to obey the Lord in all things, dying to self is a must. Death to self-will, and the Lord's will is done. There is nothing more significant before the Lord than this. What a pity man's heart is so deceitful; in this regard, even the *believer's* heart is no exception. Christian man always dwells on what he has obeyed, thus priding himself on how tenderly he has loved the Lord. Yet does he realize how very much he has *not* obeyed? May believers be granted more grace to consider more of the things which they either have not obeyed or do not obey. Unfortunately, people usually let what they have obeyed fill their thoughts. They regard what they have not obeyed and will not obey as things unnecessary, legalistic, extreme, or exclusive. May the Lord shed His light on such believers that they may realize that behind these excuses lies the fact of disobedience. How strange that people are often more rigid on things they have obeyed but very compromising on things they have not obeyed. Were they to know the Lord's heart, they would not be in such a situation. Nevertheless, it is hard to bear the cross without first sitting down and counting the cost.

3. *A Righteous Christian*   Before we trusted in the Lord Jesus we were dead in sins and transgressions. How could we know what being righteous is? After we are born again, however, we gradually come to know the degree of God's holiness and goodness. Young believers have a danger, which is derived from the new knowledge of the regenerated life. Wherein is the danger? Being over-righteous! Demanding too much righteousness from people. What does this mean? Under the new light they are in, they can clearly distinguish good from evil, right from wrong. They will then use their own spiritual understanding to measure other people. During this period they are angry at the conduct and behavior of those nominal believers. They are quick to condemn the slightest fault. Why should

so-and-so do such a thing? This becomes their usual criticism. Believers who profess to stand for righteousness often fall short themselves of the deeper work of God's grace. Had they more progress in the way of God and were they more deeply taught by the Spirit of God, they would be more lenient towards people.

The Lord Jesus in the Sermon on the Mount has sounded a certain note on this very point. Believers should not demand righteousness of other people. The Lord calls to us not to fret over those who unrighteously defraud us, beat us, force us and oppress us. His command and teaching is for us to endure and to repay them with what they do not deserve. Believers ought not demand righteousness nor should they dispense only righteousness (since righteousness is merely paying what is deserved). They are to be perfect as the heavenly Father is perfect, for He sends rain on the just and unjust alike. Let the children of God be careful lest people say Christians open their mouths only to hurt others. Christians should be strictly righteous towards *themselves* but be exceedingly lenient towards *other people*. We should give to all what they righteously deserve. This is righteousness. We should not ask for anything that people would legally have to give. This is graciousness. To be righteous towards self but to be lenient towards others involves great loss. Yet it is the road that leads to our reigning with Christ.

4. *The Manifestation of Life* The manifestation of a person's true life depends not only on a few crises but on the minute things of daily living as well. To know his spiritual measure, do not look at how he expounds the Scriptures in the pulpit, neither at how he behaves

in the assembly of the saints, nor at his public life; but look at his daily frowns and laughs, his daily words and deeds. In the early stage of Christian living, a person is full of pretension. His love, faith, patience and so forth are mostly forced. Such virtues are external. They are not the results of the work of God in his heart. For this reason, he may be able to act and perform before men, but in his private life his real self will be exposed.

In such circumstances, one lacks a genuine hatred of sins. How do we know? By looking at his heart intention. He will deeply regret and feel sorrowful when his minor faults are known to others. But if these are not known to men, his sorrow before God will be greatly lessened. It is best for a believer in such a state as this not to try to save "face." Let him go before God, confess the hatefulness and ugliness of self. By the power of the Holy Spirit let him draw upon the great finished work of the cross to put self to death that the life of God may live in him. Let him work with the Holy Spirit daily, and learn how in all things to acknowledge Him. Should anyone confess that he lives in Christ and yet he is unable to manifest the Lord's life in the many small things of the day, he needs to go to God and ask to have his real condition revealed to him.

5. *Contentment*   Contentment is a Christian virtue. Offering all to God is the first step to acquiring this virtue. Those who take God as their all possess a contented heart. Believers who long for the world cannot help but look for vainglory. But the vainglory of the world can never satisfy man's heart. No amount of fame can make a believer feel content for a single day.

Blessed are they who know the Lord Jesus as their all. Unless we ascend with the Lord Jesus and realize the emptiness of the things under the sun, we too are prone to mind the things on earth. If we are not enlightened by the Holy Spirit who causes us to understand that all which we have in Christ is eternal and real, we also will covet earthly things. Praise God, those who believe have Christ as their treasure.

6. *Hiddenness* The saints of God do not seek vainglory. We ought to hide in God. All who look for fame will be wounded by the devil. How secure and restful are those who hide in the hand of the Lord. It is abnormal for saints to seek after the glory of the world. Those who love the Lord do not desire greatness in the world. Nevertheless, so many among the believers in the Church bear secretly in their hearts the desire for high places and lofty titles. The true test for them lies not in the world but in the Church!

How wise is our Lord. He foreordains us to be called brothers and not by other titles. Sadly, many among the brethren seek to be *big* brothers. Except we allow the Holy Spirit to work into us the spirit of the cross, we shall not be exempt from possessing the evil desire for fame.

Many think the world can only be found in the world. Who knows that the world is in the Church, even in the hearts of believers! Those who have not died to the world are not freed from such base desire. Only when saints are truly joined to the Lord in His death are they dead to the world in heart.

Not seeking after vainglory is a matter of the heart.

If the Lord wills to see us in exposed places we should be willing and not draw back. Sadly, though, the fame which we get is often sought after by us. We covet in our hearts a great name for ourselves. Were we to rest in God's hand and to seek the pleasure of God alone, disregarding the judgment of men, we would find the place in which God has put us always the best place. This is the state and condition of heart at which the Lord wants us to arrive. To be hidden is not drawing back, nor is hiddenness used by us as a subtle camouflage for fame. It is not hiding somewhere externally, but is a resting inwardly in the bosom of God.

7. *Policy* This is the age of commerce. In the realm of commerce everything is conducted on the basis of policy. How sad that believers are also contaminated with this stratagem. We ought to know the difference between *truthfulness* and *policy*. There is a distance of heaven to earth between our truly loving people and our loving as a policy. Whoever truly loves loves from his heart; whoever loves out of policy loves only from his head. True love is the outflow of inward reality, whereas love out of policy is a forced external appearance. It is natural for a spiritual Christian to love truthfully, for his inside and outside agree; but to love on the basis of policy is manufactured because the inward and the outward disagree.

The behavior of a carnal Christian is mainly governed by policy. His conduct is not natural for it is not the outflow of inward reality. It is controlled by his fear of criticism or his desire for approval. Using brotherly love as an example, we see that a carnal Christian's expression of such love does not flow from real love but is manipulated to court the pronouncement of spirituality upon him by his brethren. Alas, many loves are fake. May the Lord deliver us from such pretension.

What Paul says in 1 Corinthians 13 penetrates deeply to the heart of our thoughts and intents. Such a great act as giving our body to be burned has the possibility of being without love. For it can be an act of policy, not one of truthful love. Hence the apostle judges it on this wise: "it profiteth me nothing" (v.3). Love out of policy takes care of the appearance, yet heart and mouth do not agree. It is putting on a facade, and is void of the work of God's grace. This is a deceiving of self and of others. It truly is the wiles of Satan.

Let us see that such love, generated as it is by policy, cannot endure long. With the passing of time, the real condition within will be exposed. Such forced love will not help one's spiritual life one whit. Let us rely on the cross of Christ to eliminate all such evils in heart. Let us truly love: "Let us not love in word, neither with the tongue; but in deed and truth" (1 John 3.18).

8. *Knowledge and Judging*   Judging is forbidden in the Scriptures (see Matt. 7.1). Under no circumstances should God's saints criticize. Too many Christians nowadays become their brothers' judges. We frequently hear that Christians are most critical. This seems to be a common disease among today's believers. We should ask the Lord to set watches over our mouths.

Judging is connected with man's knowledge. He who knows little tends to judge more. And he whose mind is too clear is also prone to judge. Anyone who judges quickly based on hearsay without knowing the real situation is thoughtless. Everybody has his secret. How can we possibly know all? It is very unfair to criticize before knowing all things. Let us not judge others, since we do not have the full facts. Even if we seem to possess full knowledge, we still have the possibility of some misunderstanding somewhere. Always remember how sorrowful *you* are when *you* are misunderstood and unjustly judged. Recall the untold pains of your own heart, for the people who judged you were those who also thought they had all the facts. Who knows but what there are still hidden causes. If you too have suffered under another's judging, why do you too give sufferings to other people?

Alas, oftentimes Bible knowledge aids criticism. The more head knowledge, the severer the judging. What does it profit a man to have such kind of knowledge? What is gathered from books and collected in the brain are often used as criteria for making criticism. The clearer a person is in Bible doctrines, the sterner may be his criticism of others.

The Lord has not appointed us as judges. He who judges shall be judged at the judgment seat of Christ. He who takes pleasure in censuring others without first examining himself will not be accepted by God. Let us never try to tell others God's will, for He himself shall lead them. Since God is able to lead you, He is well able to lead them too. You should not condemn your brother because he does what you disapprove of as definitely not being God's will. God is responsible for judging that brother's works and deeds. You need not hold yourself responsible.

Frequently God has already forgiven, but men are still condemning. It would appear as though men are more righteous than God! May we not fall into such error. If the Lord is patient with a brother, why can we not be patient? Let us not uncover in another the trangression which God himself has already covered. What good will it be to continue to denounce people? It does not edify men, and it is harmful to our own self, for we forget how gracious God has treated us.

In this difficult time, what the children of God need is not your criticism but your tender love. Do not aggravate their tears and pains by the untoward use of your knowledge. May we use the wine of joy and the oil of the Holy Spirit to bind up the wounds of our neighbors. May we comfort instead of judge people.

9. *Quietness* I notice a lack among today's believers: they talk too much and fail to "study to be quiet" (1 Thess. 4.11a). Many are too passive, and many are too active. Those who receive much grace from God usually have their heads bowed. Only those who are not deeply rooted in Jesus Christ cannot help but be flippant. "A fool hath no delight in understanding, but only that his heart may reveal itself" (Prov. 18.2). How true is this saying! A person uninstructed by God tends to show forth his own good. But if we are deeply taught in the Lord, we will say with Jeremiah, "I sat alone because of thy hand" (Jer. 15.17b).

A quiet life is usually a fragrant life. If we speak less, what we speak will be more powerful. Talkativeness is a point of leakage in one's spirituality. Concerning the Holy Spirit the Lord Jesus declared: "He shall glorify me: for he shall take of mine, and shall declare it unto you. ... for he shall not speak from himself" (John 16.14,13b). A man full of the Holy Spirit has this kind of life. He will not tell anything which is not received from the Lord. Not a single word will be spoken out from himself. He does not say what he loves to say, and says it only after he has been commanded by the Lord. If we truly learn to obey the Holy Spirit in this area, our daily speech will be reduced by half! This will glorify the Lord. The Holy Spirit glorifies Him in words. What, then, should we who claim to be filled with the Spirit do?

How our natural life loves to express what we know. When those more advanced brothers and sisters teach anything of which we know just a little, we are eager to declare: "This we already know...Indeed, this is what we do!" When the Lord's servant is preaching, we are anxious to show that we are not like the others in the audience who have no knowledge about what is being preached. In actuality, though, we do not realize how much we yet do not know! A quiet life is a truly knowledgeable life!

How difficult it is to remain quiet — to say nothing and remain unmoved in heart when acclaimed by the crowd. The temptation of such a time is to add a few words directly or indirectly, propagating our own glory. How beautiful it is if we are not moved by outside circumstances but maintain a quiet spirit. How rare are those who are able to take contempt and despising with serenity without murmuring at the back. Even rarer is it to be speechless before men as well as before the Lord. This is due to the fact that the inward man is not excited.

A quiet life is to be calm in the spirit. It is not only characterized by few words but is also totally unmoved by outside things. The world may have people who are born with few words and laughs, but it has none born "quiet." They who speak little and laugh little have their hearts boiling like the rest of the people. In fact, sometimes their inside is even more turbulent. But a quiet person must be one with few words. To grit one's teeth as a means to not speak is not quietness, for his heart has already been disturbed.

Unless the cross works deeply in a man's heart, it is impossible for that one to be quiet. Only after the Holy Spirit has wrought in us the meaning of the cross will He be able to rule over us and bring in quietness. Our Lord is truly our example: when the crowd wanted to force Him to be king, he retreated to the mountain; and when He stood before Pilate, he uttered not a word (see John 6.15, and Matt. 27.11–14 or Mark 15.1–4). He made no sound outwardly, thus indicating that He had no fear within.

10. *A Day Like This* Today I am so anxious as though something has been lost. I want to depart from this place and seek comfort from gathering with other saints. How hard to spend a day like this. It is not easy to be confined in this place. But such feeling, I know, comes from the soul's excitement. O Lord, I dare not make a single move; for I know that Your Spirit is working in me to divide my spirit and soul so that my spirit may ascend and become one spirit with the Spirit of the Lord Jesus beyond the touch of the soul's excitement. It is hard to endure; yet if this is endured without

fleeing from the course set by the Lord, then the soul shall lose its influence. May the Lord enable me to be still!

11. *Never Thirsty Again* The eternally blessed Lord while on earth told us: "whosoever drinketh of the water that I shall give him shall never thirst" (John 4.14a). Faithful is the saying and worthy of all acceptance. For what the Lord gives supplies us with everlasting satisfaction. The Lord knows the nature of His gift. But, alas, many times our experiences are different. Many a time we thirst again. Do we not often experience dryness? We frequently feel unsatisfied and lacking. Yet the word of our beloved Lord never fails. What He says is true. The problem lies in us. This is due to our unbelief! If we truly believed His word, we would never thirst. The living water that He has promised us ought to moisten our parched heart and fill all our desires. The more we believe in the Lord's promises, the more His life in us will spring forth. How wicked is this evil heart of unbelief! May the Lord give us grace that we may believe Him and rest in Him. Blessed are they who know how the Lord satisfies their hearts. Blessed are they who desire nothing else!

12. *Rest* We have only one resting place, which is, our Lord himself—"Rest in the Lord" (see Ps. 37.7a). If we try to rest in our environment, knowledge, health, feeling or even our spiritual experience, we shall soon see their changeableness, and thus we suffer defeat. All these are shaking foundations. Thank the Lord, *He* is our resting place. Although we cannot rest in anything else, we can rest in Him. He is our secured High Tower.

We rest in Him because of His great love. He loves us, and His love is "eternal" and "to the end" (see John 13.1). This love caused Him to come down from heaven, to be crucified for us, to be raised up from the dead, to ascend back to heaven, intercede for us, prepare a place for us and to come back again at some future appointed time. How amazing is this love! Human tongues cannot describe such love. Having such a loving God love us, is there any reason not to rest in Him? Whatever may happen, we need not be troubled and become anxious. We should rest.

Also, we rest in the Lord because of His wisdom. He never miscalculates. He knows how to arrange things and to proceed. Whatever happens to us has already been considered by His wisdom. He knows how all things work together for good to those who love Him. In spite of all this, we often imagine we have reached the end. There is nothing we can do, and our hearts are troubled. Yet the Lord is not like us. He knows He holds the whole world in His hands. He knows how to plan even small things for us. Why then be troubled? Is He not all-wise?

Furthermore, we rest in the Lord because of His almighty power. His arms never fail. The greatness of His power is unthinkable. Whatever He decides to do, He has the power to fulfill it. He has the power to deliver His children. He has the power to destroy the works of the devil. He forever triumphs. This power now works for us. Therefore, let all trembling and feeble brethren rest boldly in the Lord. For this powerful Lord is our Father. May the Lord cause us to look to Him and to rest in times of trouble. May we believe in His love, wisdom and power, and thereby be free from unnecessary anxieties.

13. *Self-proclamation* Self-proclamation is to place ourselves in an inappropriate position. This is both a danger to young believers and a snare to old saints. Only after the cross has done its practical work in a man's heart can he be weaned from the desire of proclaiming himself and be willing to let other people be glorified. Only then can he silently stay in God's quiver and sheath. Not for a moment can a Christian's life be separated from the cross, for the Holy Spirit of God uses it to deal with us and to expose our corruption. After a saint has been so trained by God, he knows in experience his own unworthiness. Henceforth, not only will he have no desire to advertise himself but he also will consider such action as shameful. God has already revealed to him his real condition. The more a person knows himself the less that one will promote himself. What is regrettable is that we do not know ourselves. We ought to see light in God's light (cf. Ps. 36.9).

There are different degrees of self-proclamation. Some blow their own horns before men; others subtly praise themselves. Yet all have the same desire in them. Some declare themselves out of pride—esteeming themselves more excellent than others; some announce themselves out of jealousy—uplifting themselves to be equal. All these are but the works of the flesh. Even if there be better motives than these, all nevertheless fall into the snare of self. It seems to be the common sin of men to worship the created rather than giving glory to the Creator. In the event of God giving glory and honor to Christian men, it more than likely will arouse Christian man's heart to indulge in hero worship. How much more attention will be drawn to self-proclamation! Not to mention the harm done to others, the fact of his own spiritual barrenness will also be a foregone conclusion. Though there may be some external success, he has already lost ground in the matter of spiritual warfare. Nowadays, alas, how countless are circular letters and reports! The Lord have mercy on me not to judge. Nonetheless, few give glory to God! In many so-called offerings of praise to Him, there is more the praise of men, even the praise of self mixed in with it! Many a time our hearts look for God as well as men to praise us.

In many works, God is placed way behind. We wonder who is ruling. In any case, self-proclamation cannot be reasonably justified. When we were babes in Christ, did we not do this? How happy we were being praised and known! May the Lord enable us to know ourselves so that we may learn to be quiet and hidden.

14. *Imperfect* The Lord Jesus Christ aims at our perfection: "that he might sanctify it [the Church], having cleansed it by the washing of water with the word, that he might present the church to himself a glorious church, not having spot or wrinkle or any such thing; but that it should be holy and without blemish" (Eph. 5.26–27). Such is the expectation and determination of the Lord. How truly far short we are from this goal! True, we press on daily; nevertheless, how far away we still are from the end. The Lord wants us to be perfect, and the world also watches to see if we are perfect.

Without perfection, we cannot please Christ. Without perfection, we are not able to attract souls. It goes without saying that we have made progress since we first believed. Yet are there still many tiny defilements and spots in our character and conduct? "Dead flies cause the oil of the perfumer to send forth an evil odor" (Eccl. 10.1a). How many are these dead flies! We frequently comment: "He truly loves the Lord, but his temper is not too good"; or, "she truly is zealous, but she is somewhat proud." How very easy to detect the dead flies in the oil of others. May we come to realize how many kinds of dead flies are in our own oil. May the Lord open our eyes that we may see.

Sometimes when we are helping and saving people, our hearts are filled with the love of Christ but after a little while, we grow disturbed and become jittery. Or else, immediately after we have been used by the Lord to deliver and edify others, we steal the glory to ourselves. There may be times after we have labored diligently abroad—even unto death—that in returning home we have lit up the fire of hell because we found ourselves not appreciated. On occasion we have said that we are not trying to broadcast the faults of another, but we then relate them so that other people can pray for him! We may love the brethren according to the Lord's teaching, but other people we treat coldly and harshly, excusing ourselves with the explanation that they are separate from us. In the daily living of the saint, how many are the dead flies indeed!

All who truly seek after holiness should recognize these flies. Satan—or Beelzebub, which means, "king of flies"—always tries to put flies in our lives, causing us to fail in success. This really is indicative of imperfection. We should confess our failure before the Lord and ask Him to wash us constantly with the water and the word. What is regretful is that the flesh is unwilling. We ought to resist Satan and restore the ground formerly yielded up to him so that we may not be contaminated by his uncleanness. Let us seize the little foxes which spoil the vineyards (see S.S. 2.15a); let us purge the old leaven (see 1 Cor. 5.6-7); let us get rid of the little folly that would outweigh wisdom and honor (see Eccl. 10.1b) — in order that we may become perfect as the heavenly Father is perfect (see Matt. 5.48).

15. *The Believer's Giving* "Then Mordecai bade them return answer unto Esther, Think not with thyself that thou shalt escape in the king's house, more than all the Jews. For if thou altogether holdest thy peace at this time, then will relief and deliverance arise to the Jews from another place...: and who knoweth whether thou are not come to the kingdom for such a time as this?" (Esther 4.13-14) Each time I read this, I am deeply stirred. At that time the Jews, the brethren of Esther, were in a most precarious situation. They all could soon be slaughtered by their enemies. Except for Esther, there was probably no one else who could save them. The warning Mordecai gave to Esther is truly a warning to all who are capable of helping other brethren. To deliver the Jews was God's purpose. He had determined to save His people for He would not allow them to be annihilated. God honored Esther, calling her to be the instrument of deliverance to the Jews. But if Esther failed God, He would be forced to choose another vessel of

deliverance. But Esther would miss the glory of working with God as well as the joy which would come from helping people. "Then will relief and deliverance arise to the Jews from another place." Nowadays God's children have many needs. They not only have spiritual but also material needs. Many of God's servants and maids are in poverty because they forsook all for the Lord and "went forth, taking nothing of the Gentiles" (3 John 7).

"God shall supply every need" (Phil. 4.19), for He will not let those who trust in Him be put to shame. This is His will and His way.

Now God chooses His working vessel, His channel of water. He honors you and grants you the glory of assisting Him. Giving is not loss. There is nothing to boast of if you give. Rather, it shows how God honors you and is willing to use you. This is your glory. May we not despise this kind of glory. "Then will relief and deliverance arise to the Jews from another place." If you fail to do what God calls you to do, do you think His hand will be tied, that He is unable to do anything else? Not at all. He has His "another place." He will be forced to find another person, but *you* will miss the opportunity of assisting Him. In essence, you despise God's esteem. You rebel against His good will towards you. You are a failure to God, and you nearly cause Him to fail too. Even so, He has rich resources. Initially He honors men by calling them to participate in His works and ministry. If men fail, can He not send ravens and dispense manna from heaven?

God always has "another place." What is lamentable is that we fail to obtain the joy and glory of working with Him. All who maintain close communion with the Lord know the value of working with Him. All who have the mind of Christ sense the Lord's despair and pain. If the Lord could use His word upon us to divide our spirit and soul, thereby giving us ascendant experience, we would know how to sympathize with Him and how to take His interest as ours. We would not be unconcerned about what God has done through His other children. Let us always remember this: "who knoweth whether thou are not come to the kingdom for such a time as this?" Today God gives you abundance in order that you can also give abundantly.

16. *Busy* The word "busy" on the lips of believers is quite prevalent these days. However, the burden the Lord has given us is light and easy. He has not asked us to bear that which we are unable to bear. It is very important for us to remember this, for this can give us many comforts! Many Christians are always saying, I am busy, very busy! They are busy from dawn to dusk. They labor incessantly without any leisure. Their burdens look most heavy. I am not simply talking about ordinary believers in their daily works; I am also talking about those of us who work directly the work of God.

It is definitely not the Lord's will for His children to be so busy that they have no time to commune and converse with Him in solitude. Most certainly it is not God's mind for His workmen to go fishing the whole day without there being time set aside to mend their nets. Allow me to say most frankly, many "busynesses" are busy for nothing. Let every child of God stop and think: Is it true that if I were not so busy, the work would not be done?—that people would not be able to live? I suspect that many busynesses can be spared. They are unnecessary. We get involved either through the instigation of Satan or by the demand of circumstances. How cruel are these two masters—environment and Satan. The wiles of the Enemy are either to pull or to push. If he is not able to pull us from going forward, he will push us to walk faster. Perhaps, indeed, many of our busynesses are instigated by him. Neither, it would seem, does the demand of circumstances give us a moment's rest. Every hour and every minute it beckons us to work. How could we have allowed circumstances to manage us so? Yet I know many times we *can* spend our day without being busy. For much of our busynesses are stirred by circumstances, and therefore they are unnecessary.

The best guide by which to work is the will of God. Are all of the works you do in the day ordered by Him? Otherwise, why do you do them? What keeps us busy are not big and important things, but sundry, small things. Are these ordered by God for us to do? If we were to examine carefully everything we do in a given day most likely we would reduce many items from our daily agenda!!

Generally speaking, when we are busy with many things, our hearts tend to be troubled. We lose our inward tranquillity. "Martha was cumbered about much serving" (Luke 10.40a). The Lord wants us to keep that inward tranquillity in Him. He does not want us to lose the good part. We ought to understand that it is not much work which shall induce the Lord's reward.

Reward is given to those who faithfully do the will of God. What is the profit if we do that which is not God's will? Not to be cumbered is not a shunning of responsibility; rather, it is an enabling of us to have more time to commune with the Lord and to please Him more. In any case, to be busy working cannot be compared with our being busy praying. Substitute busyness with prayer, and more will be accomplished.

17. *Offer Secular Things* Every believer should be involved in personal witnessing, though not all will be occupied exclusively with preaching. In the case of those who do the Lord's work, naturally what they do daily should be the work of the Lord. Ordinary believers must go out to work in order to feed themselves and their families. Those who truly serve the Lord know that what they do is His work and one day they shall receive their reward. Hence, the more they work, the greater shall be their interest and joy. Ordinary belivers know that what they do are earthly jobs. They are fully aware how these works are vain and transient. But they must work to feed themselves and their families. They therefore have no joy in their works. How sad!

Sadder still are the sisters in the Lord. Many of them love the Lord very much and are willing to serve Him. Their hearts burn with the thought of working for Him. But they already have families. They are either wives or mothers. They have many things to do at home. Housework takes up most of their time. They are troubled because out of love they wish they could serve the Lord and yet they cannot. Furthermore, those who labor for the gospel often sense the presence of the Lord because what they do is the work of God. But those who are involved in taking care of secular matters— whether hearing the cries of children, the noise of the crowd and the clanging of the kitchen, or even quietly sitting in the office—seem to find it difficult to sense God's presence. Nonetheless, is not God Father to all who believe in Him? "Father"—how lovely and tender is this word! How He cares for us. Those who preach the gospel are His children, so are those His children who manage mundane things. He gives the same care to the secular jobbers as to the evangelists.

In order to meet God in all kinds of work and to have His presence, we must recall again and again this word: "whatsoever ye do, work heartily, as unto the Lord, and not unto men" (Col. 3.23). This is the good news preached by the apostles. Let us praise God for He not only accepts those who work directly for Him but also is pleased with whatever works His other children do for Him. "Whatever ye do": All legitimate works —as long as they are unmixed with sins—we may do as unto the Lord. Therefore the mothers who nurse the babes may count their labor as done unto the Lord. The wives who manage homes can likewise so reckon their work. Those who are employed in offices and serve their employers can also consider themselves as working unto the Lord. Let us not forget that whatever we do is done as unto the Lord. During work, let us tell Him: "O Lord, I do this as unto You! For Your sake I am doing it." This will sanctify all our works. We may serve God in all things. However, if the Lord calls you to serve Him exclusively and directly, you ought to obey.

18. *Alone* Frequently God's children are lost in the crowd. Hence they lose their communion with God. How many things disturb us in our daily life. How much they affect us spiritually. Much communication with men and less communion with God is a fatal blow to a believer's spiritual walk. People ask me how they can sense more of the Lord's presence and know more of His love? My answer is: Commune often with the Lord. You should be alone in a place and meditate on His word and work. Ask Him what He requires of you. Tell Him your heartache as well as your inner desire. Be alone in His presence, lift up your head and listen to His still, small voice. Look at His lovely face. At least during half an hour each day (the more the better) you should leave your homefolks and friends, take your Bible, walk alone in the desert or sit quietly on a hillside. Alone in one place or in a room, kneel before the Lord and quietly commune with God the Father and the Lord Jesus His Son. Thus shall we have His power manifested to us. His presence, His love, His glory and His holiness will daily become more and more a reality to us.

I notice the great lack among modern believers is to be quiet in the presence of God. Christians lay so much stress on social intercourse—in chatting with people—that they forget to commune with God. It is best we can say with the prophet Jeremiah, "I sat alone because of thy hand" (Jer. 15.17b). High flying birds do not fly in flocks. The healthier and stronger a saint's spiritual life is, the less he joins the crowd. He is not able to walk at the same pace. It is as if apart from the Lord he has no companion. This is a kind of sanctified aloneness! Such a person is like the one described by the psalmist:

"a sparrow that is alone upon the housetop" (Ps. 102.7). There is a kind of tranquillity, serenity and peace here which is unknown to the world. The presence of the Lord is most evident. The person's word, thought and action seem to carry "heaven" in them. People see him as out of the world, a heavenly man, for he breathes the uncontaminated air of heaven. He is so separated from the world that his holy living possesses unusual power. Wherever he goes, he carries with him an atmosphere that touches people.

Yet this aloneness is not to be confused as any refusal to live with men as was often the case with monks of old. Though the spirit of such people alone differs from that of the world, they love more and are more lovable because they know more of God. They are not trying to single themselves out as superior. In spirit they are like heavenly people; but in the body of Christ they are full of the love and gentleness of the Lord. Daily they set apart a time for spiritual growth. How blessed is such a life!

19: *Love the Lord* Our Lord is worthy to be loved and respected. Love must find expression, and consecration is the first and the last of love's expressions. With love, there is always something to offer. What today's saints lack is more love and deeper consecration. However, with love there is always consecration, yet with offering there is not necessarily love. It is still possible to give one's body to be burned and have not love (see 1 Cor. 13.3). Each external deed should be motivated by inner affection, otherwise it is only an outward act and signifies that the first love has already left. This is unacceptable to the Lord. In our service to Him may we be constrained by the love of Christ to offer ourselves and possessions to Him. "Let us not love in word, neither with the tongue; but in deed and truth" (1 John 3.18). Weak is our love if this be only in heart with no outside expression.

The way believers manage their wealth is a thermometer by which to measure their love towards the Lord. What percentage of your possessions is used for the Lord? How much do you use for yourself, for your family and your children? By answering these questions, you should know how much you love the Lord. Is His work less important than our daily fare and our children's tuition? Do we offer all our living to please the Lord or offer only that which is left? Although many believers are poor, there are still some who are quite rich. If there is love towards the Lord, even the poor have their "two mites" (see Mark 12.42 and Luke 21.2). How can you fail to express your love even with but "two mites"? As to the rich, I am afraid their offerings are but the crumbs which fall from their tables. Who of us truly realizes that our Lord being so rich became so poor for us? We must therefore be poor for His sake. No one will lack food and clothing as a result of his helping in the Lord's work.

If those rich children of God really love the Lord they could supply the need of His temple without having to make any sacrifice in their daily living. If they fervently love Him, their money that lies idle in the banks could be circulated for the Lord's use. They would even be willing to deny many of their daily enjoyments in order to give pleasure to God's heart. Yet how few are those who know the joy of offering! And not just ordinary believers, but also God's workmen, who may not receive much—these, too, like the Levites in the Old Testament period who gave their one-tenth, should not be deprived of such an experience of love. Although what we do is the Lord's work and what we use is God's money, that which we offer with tears is not despised by the Lord. (However, let us be careful to give only for the Lord's use. Nowadays there are many so-called churches and institutions which have left the truth of the Lord. What they preach is not the gospel; what they do is not in one accord with God's will. Let us be careful in giving lest it not be acceptable to God, but promotes heresy instead.) Finally, let me say that in case we bury our money, time and energy, we shall regret this in eternity for we have not used them for the Lord.

20. *Meditate on Christ* The four Gospels record the perfect life of the Lord Jesus. Matthew presents Him as "king"; Mark, as "servant"; Luke, as "man"; and John, as "God." In reading the gospels we usually commit one mistake, which is, that we notice only the words and the deeds of Christ. Truly His words and deeds are powerful enough to engross our souls. Nevertheless, we fail to see Christ himself in a way we ought to see. The reason for studying the record of His works and speech is for the sake of knowing the *living* Christ. For this, we must spend time in meditation. First meditate on God's revealed record, and then meditate on the Christ it has revealed.

We should sit quietly, open the Bible, read a portion of the beautiful life of our Lord, then meditate on His wisdom, grace, patience, love, beauty, gentleness, tenderness and sympathy. We should ponder Him till His life leaps from the page and our hearts are burned with longing for Him. How precious, lovely and gentle He is. We ought to muse on Him till His tender deeds appear before our eyes and draw us deeply. It will cause us to long for Him. Unless we taste His love and gain Him wholly, we are at a loss. We should consider His works till our own lives are characterized by His kindness and grace.

We all are familiar with the wisdom of the Lord Jesus in the answer He gave about the origin of authority. We are familiar, too, with His marvelous solution to this matter of paying tax to Caesar. In truth, all his actions are full of love. May we know our Savior more.

21. *Thoughtfulness* Rudeness does not belong to godly life. Before a believer experienced the abundant grace of God in his life, he had many rough traits. He was inconsiderate, did not think of others' need, and had no sympathy towards people's problems. This has been a common fault among the saints. Even most spiritual saints at times fail to be thoughtful.

All who are faulty here show that they are unable to exercise full control over their mind. Carelessness is a sign of the lack of such control. In the case of such persons, their mind is scattered and confused. Their thoughts become tangled up, and they have no power to concentrate. Because of this, they tend to forget and are inconsiderate in their dealings with others.

Paying too much attention to one's own self is also a major reason for negligence in this area. In order to benefit himself, such a thoughtless person disregards the needs of others. When people are asleep, he makes noises without any thought that he might be disturbing others (sometimes, in fact, these may even be sounds of prayer and Bible reading!). In gatherings, he causes people to have to wait till he has concluded his private affairs. To protect his own name, he slanders others; to preserve his own profit, he defrauds other people. Due to a lack of the spirit of the cross in his life, he consciously or unconsciously neglects other people and is not thoughtful of them. Sometimes he may do things out of an honest heart; nonetheless, how these actions of his embarrass people!

Frequently we may deem our thoughtlessness as being a characteristic of straightforwardness and something without guile. But rudeness is not a fruit of the Holy Spirit. What a saint should do is to seek to be considerate in all things, be thoughtful to men, sympathetic to their problems, and cause no embarrassment to anyone.

The cross of the Lord and the Holy Spirit have the power to refine, causing the roughest of us to be gentle. Except one is truly dead to the self-life, he is not able to be considerate in all things and thoughtful towards all men. Only when dead to self will he not think of his own right and be willing to suffer to seek the other's profit. We should exercise our will to control our mind so that we will not be negligent and forgetful of other people's needs. The principle at work in us should always be: "So then death worketh in us, but life in you" (2 Cor. 4.12). The spirit of the cross must indeed be our standard!

22. *Prayer and Desire* Prayer is the expression of our heart desire towards God. The Bible records many prayers answered because they were all offered as definite heart desires. Without desire there is no need to pray. If what we ask for really comes out of our heart, our prayer will more frequently be answered. Due to our lack of singleness of desire, our prayer sounds more like clanging cymbals.

The greatest danger to prayer is to pray elaborately and traditionally. Such traits increase in public prayers. Actually, nine out of ten such eloquent prayers are empty. They are most likely offered for men to hear rather than for God. Many a time these are offered with noble sentiment, earnest voice and pleasant tone; but they are for human consumption. God will neither hear nor answer such prayers. Praying without heart desire is playing with God. It is abominable in His sight. Is it not true that even in private prayer we often use words more out of habit than out of heart? Because these words sound so familiar the heart does not respond at all. Such prayer is really a waste of time. It is worse than unprofitable.

Those who truly know God and His majestic holiness will not pray so. As we come before Him with a pure heart, realizing who is on the other side, we dare not be false. As a matter of fact, our prayer can never exceed the moving of the Holy Spirit. Whatever goes beyond that is hypocritical. Hence, when praying, it is best to let the Holy Spirit put what we should pray for in our spirit. And thus we will not offend God. Learn to be true before Him. Pray a short prayer rather than pray untruthfully.

This point needs to be underlined in relation to intercessory prayer. Many such prayers are more in the nature of repayment of debts. For this reason, there is no heart desire; it is only a going through the motion. People without real love are unable and unfit to intercede for others. Only after we sense the other's need as our own can we intercede with a true heart. Then are we able to pray faithfully. Without love we can only intercede vocally. We should be more sympathetic towards, and more united with, other people. May we henceforth pray with heart as well as with lips. May our prayers ascend as incense to God.

23. *Holiness and Hardness* Christians ought to be both undemonstrative as well as affectionate. Because they know only heavenly things and desire nothing but the Lord Jesus, they are most undemonstrative. On the other hand, since they do not choose whom to love, they love all the brethren — including the loving and the unloving; they even love their enemies; and hence, they are the most affectionate.

Holiness is the goal of a believer. A slight deviation may nonetheless turn our holiness into another's stumbling block. In our human experience holiness can frequently turn into hardness! Believers who seek for holiness often embarrass people. The holier they become, the more things their eyes condemn, and the more that unloving discussions and criticisms follow. The holiness of him who has not experienced deeply the grace of God impresses people as stoical and brainless. Such a person cannot help others. He only draws down denunciation upon himself.

People like to regard themselves as upholding God's standard and bearing a good testimony to His truth. They forget that holiness is of God. We should never forget that we are but men; we ought always to acknowledge this; we should not imagine that we are as holy as God. God's holiness is awesome and irreproachable. Though we are saved and regenerated, we still are human. We should "imbibe" the holiness of God and make it ours, for such holiness is the "life mark" of the Lord Jesus. He is the Holy One who became flesh. On the one hand, in spirit He is separated from sinners. When on one occasion Peter saw Him, he cried out, "Depart from me, for I am a sinful man, O Lord" (Luke 5.8b). On the other hand, though, He is a friend of sinners. He sympathizes with publicans and prostitutes who are despised by the world. He pities them and comforts them. Just as the first-mentioned aspect of His life reveals His holiness, so this latter aspect shows forth His holiness too. He is not unapproachable, nor is He hard.

The holiness of a believer can and ought to be something very beautiful. It must not degenerate into hardness so as to court fear rather than respect and approachableness. As a matter of fact, hardness is never holiness! These two are vastly different. Holy, yes, but this refers to how one deals with one's own self; for self, there is no fear of being strict. To be empty of self-pity is a hallmark of the way of the cross. Towards other people, however, there is need to love and to be sympathetic. Though God is holy, He balances His holiness with grace. We may be holy, but let us not be hard as wood or cold like ice. God does not save us to be unhuman. On the contrary, because we have fallen into an unhuman state, He saves us that we may be human once again. For this cause, though we may appear most undemonstrative, we nonetheless are to be most affectionate.

A truly holy life is not void of the virtues of gentleness, peace and mercy. Just as in the manner that the shepherd tends his foolish sheep, so in like manner ought we to treat all people. A life poured out is a fruitful life. Hardness sends people away, but mercy melts hearts and causes them to travel together on this heavenly path.

24. *When God's Grace Manifests Itself Most*　The grace of God towards us never changes, though our feeling towards His grace may vary according to time. In fact, His grace never ceases, but our enjoyments of it always differ. To be in want is the primary factor for enjoyment of grace. The more we are in need the more precious we appreciate grace. We will never consider God's supply to be grace if we sense no lack.

Saints commit one error. We think we need God's grace only at the time we were yet sinners. It is true that through God's grace we are saved. Yet throughout our life after we are saved we still need the grace of God. Indeed, there is not a moment in our Christian walk when we are not under His grace. God forgave our sins by letting the judgment of our sins fall upon His Son, our Lord Jesus. As we believed in Him, we were saved. Such grace is truly great. But how deceitful is our heart! As we proceed on the Christian pathway (and perhaps the Lord has even given us grace to cause us to win many victories), we somehow attribute the glory of victory to ourselves, thinking that we are quite good. Although the grace of God remains the same, we in this situation do not appreciate Him and His grace as we should. In view of the deceitfulness of our hearts, God frequently allows us to be tempted — even sifted — by the devil.

When therefore we fail, we bemoan and hate ourselves, now concluding that, for us, again being sinful, it is not too much to expect that God will once more condemn us to death. Yet will He withdraw His grace from us? Let us realize that though our sins be great, His grace is still sufficient for us. He is willing to forgive our sins. In spite of our failure, God will not forsake us. And upon our sensing this, how grateful we become at such a time! We marvel at the greatness of His grace! Though we are irreparable sinners, yet He still dispenses grace and mercy and care. This causes us to be more grateful for God's abundant grace and to know that as a matter of spiritual fact we need His grace at every hour. Except God had continued to give grace, we would have been consumed along with the rest of the world.

To know one's sin is to understand the preciousness of God's grace. Grace causes man to be humble. There is no need of grace if one does not know himself to be a sinner — even a sinner saved by grace. To confess oneself a sinner is a humble act. When the Holy Spirit convicts us in respect of our sins, it is quite easy for us to be humble again. Yet how difficult it is for us to judge ourselves daily and reckon that in our flesh there is no good. It is not easy to persistently declare ourselves as unable to do good. How our heart seeks for glory, it considering itself capable of doing good; but we thereby forget the grace of God and the need for it. During those times when we humble ourselves and acknowledge that in Adam our life is corrupted and defiled, we look for the grace of God.

On the one hand God wants us to overcome daily; on the other hand He appears as though He wishes us to fall every day so that we may ask for grace. We stand in need of His grace in our daily living just as we need it when we sin. It is pitiful that only when our Adamic life flares up do we confess how defiled it is. Ordinarily we evaluate this old Adamic life within us differently, and hence we refuse to be humble. May we always acknowledge that nowhere in our old life and nature is there not the deep taint of sin upon it. Except for the grace of God, we should have long ago been consumed. Hallelujah, the Lord has grace!

25. *Sensitive to Sin* Although we honor the Lord's grace as great, we dare not despise, belittle or condone sin. God *hates* sin. Whether sins in the world or sins in the heart of the saints, He equally hates them. It is a glorious thing to proclaim the grace of God. We should do our best to spread the good news of His salvation by grace. But it will be defiling His grace if in preaching we misunderstand grace as condoning man's sin. Sin must be judged and forsaken in God's dealing with man both under law and under grace. For a person to love sin under the cover of grace indicates his total lack of understanding of the grace of God. "Shall we continue in sin that grace may abound?" All the redeemed should say with Paul, "God forbid!" (Rom. 6.1b,2a).

One thing troubles the faithful saints of God. People do not treat sin as sin. They invent many new terminologies to cover up sins. What is more disturbing is that believers take sin too lightly. How sad that many have gradually lost their sensitivity toward sin. I do not wish to imply by this that they have not wrestled with sin. They certainly have. A truly born-again person possesses a new nature that hates sin. And hence, they at one time must have strenuously resisted it. Yet due to more defeats than victories, they begin to excuse themselves with the thought that it is impossible to overcome sin. And as sins prevail, the accusing voice of conscience grows dimmer and dimmer. How pitiful! What a fall!

Perhaps they know the teaching of 1 John 1.9: "If we confess our sins, he is faithful and righteous to forgive us our sins, and to cleanse us from all unrighteousness." They mistakenly conceive a casual idea about the grace of God: Why worry about sinning if it can be forgiven by simply confessing? Though they may not say this audibly, they do endorse such an idea in their mind. This is the reason for the failure of many believers, in that they lose their sensitivity toward sin.

Spiritual sensitivity and physical sensation are alike in one respect: If we are wounded often and exposed to wind and frost too frequently, we become numb. Likewise, in this matter of despising or making light of sin, our conscience will become more and more cauterized. For once sin remains unconfessed and is belittled, conscience grows harder. Finally, the hatred of sin as a spiritual motion in us is so reduced that our sensitivity towards it becomes paralyzed.

Many are our failures in small things. A word of untruth here, a time of unfaithfulness there, a little unrighteousness elsewhere! All are but inches of defeat! Not that conscience does not accuse, but that we often console ourselves with the thought that these failures are insignificant. And thus we resist the accusation of conscience and harden our hearts. In so doing, we render a fatal blow to our sensitivity toward sin. Once we forego the accusation of conscience by not confessing our sin, we are unable to get rid of sin and will naturally lose the standard of God's holiness.

Let us never be afraid, however, of being oversensitive toward sin! Whenever conscience accuses let us judge ourselves and forsake our sin. Then shall our sensitivity towards it become sharper and sharper. An overcoming saint is a self-examining believer. Just as a sinner is fearful of the punishment of sins which is hell, so we believers should be afraid of the power of sin. We must be careful and not become hardened lest we lose that sensitivity. If spiritual sensitivity is lost, spiritual life dries up. He who makes light of, belittles or despises the seriousness of sin despises the grace of God. Knowing the terror of sin as well as the total inability of self opens the way for us to treasure the grace of God.

26. *Read and Pray* Each time I travel, I meet about a thousand believers, but less than three of the thousand read the Bible and pray daily. No wonder the Church is weak and the believers backslide.

"Too busy, too busy," "Busy from morning till night," "Where can I find time to read the Bible and pray?" Such are the explanations (excuses?) given by these many believers who fail in this daily spiritual exercise. Yet who of us is *not* busy in his life? It is just a matter of priority. "Too busy," but we still find time to eat three meals a day! It is not because of busyness that we do not eat and drink for a whole year. If God's children truly know that "man shall not live by bread alone, but by every word that proceedeth out of the mouth of God" (Matt. 4.4), then no matter how busy they are, they ought to at least be willing to forego one meal and set *that* time aside for Bible reading and prayer.

Are all of us really *so* busy? We have time to chat and to entertain. I am afraid that even if we did have the time we would not spend it in reading the Bible and praying!

"How can I read the Bible if I do not understand?" This is another so-called explanation I hear. Yet how can you understand if you do not read?

"How can I pray, not knowing how to pray?" Yet, how can you know how to pray if you do not pray?

The best time for reading and praying is the morning. But who can rise early and have morning watch if he is busy all the day and has to sleep in late? What does it profit to have morning watch only as a routine? By carefully observing a Christian's Bible reading and prayer life, we can tell his spiritual condition.

Let me ask, Do you have morning watch? Do you read and pray? How much time out of the day do you come to God, read the Bible and pray? What help do you derive if you know you should have morning watch, read and pray, and yet you do not practice it?

Now is the time: the end of all things is near, even at the doors (see Mark 13.29). From this day onward, may you decide to commune with God, to read and pray as the first thing you do upon rising from your bed. If you have another period of leisure in the day, use some or all of it also to commune with God by reading His word and praying to Him.

27. *Silent witness* "Jesus therefore six days before the passover came to Bethany, where Lazarus was, whom Jesus raised from the dead. So they made him a supper there: and Martha served; but Lazarus was one of them that sat at meat with him. Mary therefore took a pound of ointment of pure nard, very precious, and anointed the feet of Jesus, and wiped his feet with her hair: and the house was filled with the odor of the ointment" (John 12.1–3).

"The common people therefore of the Jews learned that he was there: and they came, not for Jesus' sake only, but that they might see Lazarus also, whom he had raised from the dead. But the chief priests took counsel that they might put Lazarus also to death; because that by means of him many of the Jews went away, and believed on Jesus" (John 12.9–11).

In these passages of Scripture we see that Martha was there at the home in Bethany, Mary was there, and Lazarus too was there. What did Martha do? As always she served the Lord. Mary did what she had always formerly done too, which was, to perform an act of consecration. What about Lazarus? What do you think he should have been doing? Martha was loved by the Lord Jesus; Mary was loved by the Lord Jesus; Lazarus too was loved by the Lord Jesus. At that time, Martha served the Lord, Mary offered to the Lord, but Lazarus was simply sitting there. Yet what was the effect of this merely sitting there? We learn from these Scripture passages that many Jews believed on the Lord Jesus that day because of Lazarus. The latter did nothing. He did not offer anything but simply sat there quietly. Yet in that simple act of sitting quietly by, God was glorified!

TITLES YOU
WILL WANT TO HAVE

by Watchman Nee

Basic Lesson Series
Volume 1 — A Living Sacrifice
Volume 2 — The Good Confession
Volume 3 — Assembling Together
Volume 4 — Not I, But Christ
Volume 5 — Do All to the Glory of God
Volume 6 — Love One Another

The Church and the Work
Volume 1 — Assembly Life
Volume 2 — Rethinking the Work
Volume 3 — Church Affairs

Take Heed
Worship God
Interpreting Matthew
Back to the Cross
The Character of God's Workman
Gleanings in the Fields of Boaz
The Spirit of the Gospel
The Life That Wins
From Glory to Glory
The Spirit of Judgment
From Faith to Faith
The Lord My Portion
Aids to "Revelation"
Grace for Grace
The Better Covenant
A Balanced Christian Life
The Mystery of Creation
The Messenger of the Cross
Full of Grace and Truth — Volume 1
Full of Grace and Truth — Volume 2
The Spirit of Wisdom and Revelation
Whom Shall I Send?
The Testimony of God
The Salvation of the Soul
The King and the Kingdom of Heaven
The Body of Christ: A Reality
Let Us Pray
God's Plan and the Overcomers
The Glory of His Life
"Come, Lord Jesus"
Practical Issues of This Life
Gospel Dialogue
God's Work
Ye Search the Scriptures
The Prayer Ministry of the Church
Christ the Sum of All Spiritual Things
Spiritual Knowledge
The Latent Power of the Soul
Spiritual Authority
The Ministry of God's Word
Spiritual Reality or Obsession
The Spiritual Man

by Stephen Kaung

Discipled to Christ
The Splendor of His Ways
Seeing the Lord's End in Job
The Songs of Degrees
Meditations on Fifteen Psalms

ORDER FROM:

Christian Fellowship Publishers, Inc.
11515 Allecingie Parkway
Richmond, Virginia 23235